# Medical Humanities

# Medical Humanities

*Edited by*

Martyn Evans
*Senior Lecturer, Centre for Philosophy and Healthcare,
School of Health Science, University of Wales, Swansea*

and

Ilora G Finlay
*Honorary Professor of Palliative Medicine,
University of Wales College of Medicine, Cardiff
Consultant, Velindre NHS Trust Oncology Centre, Cardiff
Medical Director, Holme Tower Marie Curie Centre, Penarth*

© BMJ Books 2001
BMJ Books is an imprint of the BMJ Publishing Group

First published in 2001
by BMJ Books, BMA House, Tavistock Square,
London WC1H 9JR

www.bmjbooks.com

**British Library Cataloguing in Publication Data**

A catalogue record for this book is available from the British
Library

ISBN 0-7279-1610-6

Typeset by FiSH Books, London WC1
Printed and bound by Selwood Printing Ltd., West Sussex

# Contents

List of contributors                                                    vii

Acknowledgements                                                         ix

Foreword   *John Wyn Owen CB*                                             x

Introduction   *Martyn Evans and Ilora G Finlay*                          1

**Section 1 Humanities Reflecting Society**
*Introduction*                                                            7
1   The nature and role of the medical humanities
    *David Greaves*                                                      13
2   Society, community, well-being   *Ray Pahl*                          23
3   "No appealing solution": evaluating the outcomes of
    arts and health initiatives
    *François Matarasso*                                                 36
4   Medical records as catalogues of experience
    *Anne Borsay*                                                        50

**Section 2 Patients and Professionals**
*Introduction*                                                           77
5   The consultation as Rubik's cube   *Kieran Sweeney*                  83
6   The new genetics: retelling and reinterpreting an old story
    *Deborah Kirklin*                                                   101
7   Poetry as a key for healthcare   *Gillie Bolton*                    119
8   Spirituality as an integral part of healthcare
    *Ilora G Finlay and Paul Ballard*                                   136

**Section 3 Changing Attitudes**
*Introduction*                                                          151
9   Portfolio learning: the humanities in medical education
    *Ilora G Finlay*                                                    156
10  A pragmatic approach to the inclusion of the creative
    arts in the medical curriculum   *Bernard Moxham*                   167

11 United in grief: monuments and memories of
   the Great War   *Angela Gaffney*                         177
12 Why medical humanities now?   *Jane Macnaughton*         187
13 Medical humanities: means, ends, and evaluation
   *Robin Downie*                                           204

**Section 4 Understanding Medical Knowledge**
*Introduction*                                              219
14 Validating the facts of experience in medicine
   *John Saunders*                                          223
15 The humanities' role in improving health and clinical care
   *Richard Edwards*                                        236
16 Philosophy and the medical humanities   *Martyn Evans*   250

Alphabetical list of references                             264

Index                                                       285

# List of Contributors

**Paul Ballard**
Professor of Religious Studies, University of Wales, Cardiff

**Gillie Bolton**
Writer, Research Fellow in Medical Humanities, University of Sheffield

**Anne Borsay**
Senior Lecturer in History, University of Wales, Lampeter

**Robin Downie**
Professor of Moral Philosophy, University of Glasgow

**Richard Edwards**
Professor (Emeritus) University of Wales College of Medicine, Past Director of Wales Office for Research and Development in Health and Social Care

**Martyn Evans**
Senior Lecturer, Centre for Philosophy and Healthcare, School of Health Sciences, University of Wales, Swansea

**Ilora G Finlay**
Honorary Professor of Palliative Medicine at University of Wales College of Medicine, Cardiff, Consultant at Velindre NHS Trust Oncology Centre, Cardiff, and Medical Director of Holme Tower Marie Curie Centre, Penarth

**Angela Gaffney**
Research Fellow, Centre for Advanced Welsh and Celtic Studies, University of Wales

**David Greaves**
Senior Lecturer, Centre for Philosophy and Healthcare, School of Health Sciences, University of Wales, Swansea

**Deborah Kirklin**
Co-director of the Medical Humanities Unit, Department of Primary Care and Population Sciences, Royal Free and University College Medical School

**Jane Macnaughton**
Director, Centre for Arts and Humanities in Health and Medicine, University of Durham

**François Matarasso**
Writer and Researcher on Cultural Policy, Comedia, Nottingham

**Bernard Moxham**
Professor of Anatomy, Cardiff School of Biosciences, University of Wales, Cardiff

**John Wyn Owen**
Secretary, The Nuffield Trust, London

**Ray Pahl**
Professor of Sociology, University of Essex

**John Saunders**
Consultant Physician, Nevill Hall Hospital, Abergavenny; Secretary, Committee for Ethical Affairs, Royal College of Physicians, London, and Chairman, Multicentre Research Ethics Committee, Wales

**Kieran Sweeney**
Lecturer, Institute of General Practice, School of Postgraduate Medicine and Health Sciences, University of Exeter

# Acknowledgements

This book proceeds from an invited seminar at the University of Wales, Gregynog, in April 1999, which was made possible by the generosity of the Nuffield Trust, which we gratefully acknowledge. We are indebted to all our contributors to this volume, nearly all of whom were participants at that seminar, and also to all other participants at the seminar whose contributions to discussion stimulated and enriched the material which has subsequently been developed for publication here. The seminar's success reflects also the assured chairmanship of John Wyn Owen, Secretary of the Nuffield Trust; we are grateful to him. We are indebted also to Mr David Welsh, formerly of the Nuffield Trust, for assistance, advice, and encouragement during the process of bringing the book to publication. We greatly appreciate the guidance and encouragement given us by Mary Banks, our Commissioning Editor at BMJ Books.

Finally we are grateful to our families and colleagues for their support and forbearance.

# Foreword

John Wyn Owen CB

Humanities and Medicine, Arts, Health and Well-being is one of the major current themes of the Nuffield Trust. This publication brings this theme together with some of the Trust's other priorities, particularly Policy Futures and Devolution. Doctors and other health professionals of the future will need to deal with issues of enormous complexity as medicine and health in this new millennium deal with prevention – the reduction or removal of some risks – major changes in screening technology, social engineering, control of disease, non-invasive technology and biotechnology. The Art of the Practice of the Science of Medicine was the theme of Sir David Weatherall's opening of our first conference on Humanities and Medicine which led to the Windsor Declaration.[1] Sir David explained that the art of healing versus the science of healing is a very complex issue.

The last 10–15 years have seen a change of emphasis from the whole patient and whole organs to diseases of molecules and cells. There is a concern that molecular medicine is reductionist and dehumanising. A reductionist approach to disease has led to an understanding of evolutionary biology which has shown that each human is unique. This essential phase in the development of medical knowledge has brought together medicine and biology and not separated them. We will now start putting the bits back together again. The old skills of clinical practice, the ability to interact with people, will be as vital in the new millennium as they have been in the past.

Another of the Trust's interests is the changing role of the state in health policy – globalisation and devolution. Across the world the nation-state is changing, driven by the contradictory developments of globalisation and devolution. Giddens cites the dynamics of Welsh and Scottish devolution. "Local nationalisms are a response to a globalising process that allows you to situate your identity elsewhere. The result is a more cosmopolitan state whose peoples have multiple identities. You will be able to be Scottish, British and European."[2]

In the Nuffield Trust publication *Devolution and Health*, Hazell and Jervis said: "There is scope for considerable innovation and experimentation in the different home countries, organisation management and delivery of services." The theme of humanities and medicine was identified at a meeting of the Institute of Welsh Affairs as an area for policy development which would enable Wales, using its new devolved administrative and policy instruments, to shape a distinctive agenda and which would be of wide interest. This publication is a contribution to the emerging agenda and is based on the proceedings of a meeting sponsored by the Nuffield Trust at the University of Wales at Gregynog which was led by Martyn Evans and colleagues and encourages a formal understanding of arts, humanities and social sciences together with detailed scientific knowledge, and applying both spheres of knowledge equally to the techniques of care and cure. Clinicians and patients will benefit from providing and receiving care which is founded on a more complete understanding of how people's medical conditions exist within the individual's family and cultural context.

John Wyn Owen
Secretary, Nuffield Trust
July 2000

# References and notes

1  The Declaration of Windsor. In: Philipp R, Baum M, Mawson A, Calman KC. *The humanities in medicine: beyond the millennium*. London: The Nuffield Trust, 1999: 111–14.
2  Boynton RS. The two Tonys. *New Yorker* 1997; 6 October.

# Introduction

Martyn Evans and Ilora G Finlay

This is a book about how medicine appears through the many sides of a prism, a prism consisting of human curiosity, need, attainment, compassion, and experience, among other things. Medical knowledge is a peculiarly intense, vivid and intimate field of knowledge about ourselves as human beings and inevitably it involves – we might say *embodies* – knowledge about our many aspects as human beings, both physical and psychological, both material and personal, even spiritual. As medicine concerns our physical nature, it seems well grounded in the natural sciences but our physical nature is not the whole story about us. Moreover, we are not simply physical beings with a merely *additional* psychological, personal or spiritual aspect. Our nature is one in which the personal is *integrated* with the physical, so that the natural sciences on their own cannot tell the full story even about our physical selves. Our bodily tissues inform our personal identities, appearances, motives, desires, appetites, abilities, hopes, and fears but these personal aspects of us in their turn drive what happens to us physically and exert a powerful influence over the ways in which we fall ill and the ways in which we recover our health.

The implications of this have probably always been recognised in clinical practice but they are now increasingly recognised in the official establishments of medical education, regulation, and research. We can summarise them quite briefly. Since medicine is concerned at least with responding to our illnesses, our physical incapacities and our bodily suffering, then it could not consist of the natural biological sciences alone (even if we were to set aside, for the moment, medicine's proper attention to some aspects of our psychological suffering).

That means that the intellectual resources for clinical medicine must be drawn from other sources as well, including the social and behavioural sciences and the liberal humanities disciplines such as history, literature, law, ethics and philosophy. These humanities disciplines represent distinct ways of being interested in and making sense of human experience. They are distinct ways of recording and interpreting human experience, including the experiences of health and illness, of seeking and undergoing – and, for that matter, providing – medical care. And if we take the view, above, that human nature integrates the physical and the personal, then we should expect to find that the humanities are not an (optional) addition to scientific medical knowledge but hold an *integral* place with the natural sciences at the core of clinical medicine. Together – in a sense *fused* together, if we knew how – the natural sciences and the humanities hold the resources for trying to understand and respond to the human experiences of ill health, disability, incapacity, and suffering.

This book proceeds from that fundamental recognition. It brings together wide-ranging contributors from many disciplines, including scientific medicine, that constitute our many-sided prism for looking at medicine as a practice. Each contributor will tend to look most clearly through one or other of the particular sides of the prism, though reading the book in its entirety offers a composite view of medicine refracted by the prism as a whole. Of course, different disciplines speak somewhat different languages from each other, with different interests and concerns, and vocabularies reflecting those concerns. They will tend to *see* different things in the objects they study; we might even say they have somewhat distinct objects in view, even when ostensibly looking at the same thing. So the social scientists may see roles, historians may see processes, scholars of literature may see "characters", semioticians may see signs or symbols, philosophers may see arguments, and so on.

The point is that we need not choose among these. They are all relevant and important to an understanding of the clinical encounter, the needs of physician and patient, the interests and responsibilities of the individual and society, and the models, methods and assumptions of medical science, education, research and professional organisation and practice. Moreover, the different disciplines (and their characteristic ways of seeing) can and should converse with each other about medicine and its engagement with our nature as human beings. Ideas and terms which play an important descriptive part in one discipline might be capable of being acknowledged and adapted as organising metaphors for medicine from the perspective of another discipline. (For instance, moral philosophy has already adapted the primarily literary idea of a character[1] and this might fruitfully be incorporated into both philosophical and sociological considerations of the patient–physician relationship or, more figuratively, of the structure of medical knowledge.)

Many people are now starting to talk enthusiastically about "the medical humanities", as a field of enquiry and teaching even within the already tightly-packed medical undergraduate curriculum. But there is as yet no real consensus about what "the medical humanities" means. This book tends towards the view that the humanities (including the social and behavioural sciences) are an integral part of knowledge within the disciplines of medicine and not simply a portmanteau name for the therapeutic involvement of arts activities in healthcare provision.

The book is one result of a process of interdisciplinary discussion which was begun in the University of Wales in 1995 and which, following the establishment of postgraduate teaching and research around the "integrated conception" of the medical humanities, led to an interdisciplinary residential seminar in April 1999 in mid-Wales, hosted and funded by the Nuffield Trust. The seminar brought together from across (and beyond) Wales representatives of general practice (primary care) medicine, the performing arts, pathology, sociology, palliative care medicine, medical history, philosophy, hospital medicine, medical research and arts education. The participants included the founding co-editors of the first academic journal outside the United States to be devoted to exploring the medical humanities. This book draws together essays that were generated by the seminar. It aims to equip the reader with an understanding of the extensive interplay between different disciplines as they "refract" medicine and to recognise the importance and relevance of intellectual dialogue of this kind in improving patient care.

# Section 1
# Humanities Reflecting Society

*Introduction*                                                                        7

1   The nature and role of the medical humanities                     13
2   Society, community, well-being                                           23
3   Evaluating the outcomes of arts and health initiatives          36
4   Medical records as catalogues of experience                      50

# Introduction

"The medical humanities" is an increasingly familiar phrase in present-day discussions of medical education and practice. It does not follow from this, however, that the idea is clearly understood in a widely agreed manner. This opening section of our book begins by introducing the distinctive conception of the medical humanities which unifies the contributors to this volume as a whole. The section then goes on to explore the context which gives sense and purpose to the medical humanities and in which any broad discussion of them must be located; that is, the social context in which patients live their lives and in which medical and healthcare are organised, delivered, and evaluated.

The opening contribution, by philosopher (and public health doctor) David Greaves, sets out the "integrated" conception of the medical humanities which drives this book. Following this are three discussions firmly rooting the medical humanities in their social context. Ray Pahl, a sociologist, considers the influences upon health and well-being of individuals' experiences of their roles in family and wider social groupings. François Matarasso, a professional writer working in the field of community-based initiatives in access to and encounters with the arts, reflects on the importance of evaluating the impact of community arts initiatives upon health. Finally, historian Anne Borsay invites us to consider the making and recording of the history of medicine as itself a social practice and one, moreover, which deepens our understanding of medicine's social context today.

Let us briefly introduce these discussions in a little more detail. Greaves, setting out the terms for a distinctively "integrated" conception of the medical humanities, begins by noting a crisis of confidence in modern western medicine: different responses to this see medicine as being essentially a science or as being essentially an art or as being a balance of the two. It is this last response which has generated the "medical humanities" but there is as yet no general agreement on what the idea means. Some see the medical humanities as a collection of disciplines which are identified simply by their not being natural sciences or not being either natural or social sciences or as disciplines not relying on quantitative ("counting"-type) methods or, more interestingly, as being disciplines concerned with individuals" uniqueness. All of these approaches see arts and sciences as irrecoverably *separate* aspects of medicine. The approaches differ only over where the dividing line

7

between arts and sciences should be drawn. Moreover, they all share the problems of giving humanities a residual, "left-over" status after science is established and they do not challenge or reconsider the nature of the medical enterprise.

Greaves argues for an alternative approach. We should, he says, refocus on the meaning of "the human", bringing the philosophical method of critical reflection – in effect, a responsible refusal to take unexamined assumptions or arguments for granted – to medicine. Indeed, we should integrate such enquiries within medicine itself (as in, for instance, the celebrated neurological writings of Oliver Sacks). This approach can be taken to all the scientific and humanities disciplines which together bear upon the human patient, so that they all focus appropriately on *human values* and they all employ an appropriate common method. This approach recaptures a tradition in which arts and sciences are intertwined and in which sciences, however powerful, remain orientated within a concern for human values.

The case which Greaves sets out provides the intellectual context for the other contributions to this volume. The remaining contributions in this first section then bear, in their different ways, upon the social context. Social influences upon health are generally recognised as hugely important. For instance, as Ray Pahl points out, a direct link between *social support* and health is now widely accepted – social networks may even play a role in the ability of an individual to resist infection. But in putting forward these claims, social scientists must, argues Pahl, make their contribution clear, accessible and well supported. Traditionally, medicine has regarded social scientists with suspicion, disliking the jargon of social sciences and dismissing apparently obscure claims – only to embrace them subsequently as being "obvious", whilst still resisting acceptance of their consequences. A typical example is the recognition that intervention in patients' patterns of social relationships might be desirable from the point of view of their health status. Policy makers and researchers alike face resistance to the idea of enquiries or interventions in matters of personal relationships (as distinct from other lifestyle factors such as diet).

Some societal factors, such as economic indicators, are well recognised as determinants of health; variations within such groupings (micro-social worlds) require us to recognise the influence of *relationships*. As Pahl reminds us, the idea of "community" requires caution and has to some extent been discredited; for instance, is it a self-evidently good thing if it arises out of (avoidable) adversity such as prolonged local unemployment or a history of industrial accidents? More promising, thinks Pahl, might be the idea of social networks and more particularly the idea of personal communities, meaning those people socially significant to a given individual. Again the notion of "family" requires caution in that roles and responsibilities can no longer easily be read off from the fact of familial ties, which may obscure more powerful social relationships in a more mobile society than hitherto. Friends are becoming more kin-like with regard to social support; kin more friend-like in terms of the degree of choice in associating with them. Notwithstanding these complexities, Pahl asks, how can "better" personal communities be promoted within a concern to promote health and well-being, without incurring the hazards of unjustified "social engineering"?

Some sorts of personal communities seem visibly better at promoting well-being, in particular, those communities involving emotional support. The quantity rather than the quality of social connectedness is what is important. However it is of course ludicrous to suppose that "friends" could be state provided to support or supply such connectedness, however essential it may be to well-being and health. The best option, Pahl suggests, is to encourage common activities and here the arts and humanities have a clear role: personal communities grow from common engagement in activities and those social trends that discourage people from taking part must somehow be countered. Given the variety of such activities there is no simple prescription for how they can be promoted and so far little scholarly research has been done on the subject. But since the correlation is so well recognised, the social causations involved must be explored and understood as far as possible, including the range, functions and meaning of different forms of friendship. This is the challenge that Pahl sets out for the social sciences" contribution to the medical humanities agenda.

Interventions at the social level, whether or not they are part of a larger organised strategy, need to be *evaluated* if we are to learn about them or from them. François Matarasso considers this problem in connection with gauging the health impact of community arts projects. For Matarasso, the key questions concern, put simply, how people decide what is good for them. This is no easy matter in the context of "arts and health", since even the core terms themselves need to be examined. The external *form* of art is often mistaken for its substance, he argues, and there is no general agreement even on the meaning of "health". Matarasso suggests that we view art as a set of resources through which we think about our experiences of the world and of ourselves, a method of exploration and expression. (In this, he points out, art parallels science, since both allow us to do things which can be done or said in no other way.) He notes that "health" is used sometimes to mean a set of functional norms and sometimes a variable form of experience. Both versions find their way into different instruments for assessing health, but only the second version is really amenable to the influence of encounters with the arts. As such, the arts contribute to health promotion in various ways, through a broadening and deepening of one's sense of "well-being".

If we accept this version of "health", how can arts projects be evaluated for their health impact? Matarasso distinguishes a project's aims, objectives, methods, inputs, outputs, and *outcomes* and argues that all must be taken account of in relation to agreed standards of success, defined by the consent of those taking part. Specifically, when it comes to the engagement between arts and health, it must first be determined – and not simply assumed – whether the specific health needs really are best addressed by an arts project rather than by some other kind of activity. We should, says Matarasso, choose the extent of our engagement with the arts, just as we choose the extent of our engagement with medical and healthcare. Very much in this spirit, Matarasso argues that the "bottom line" in deciding how to measure the impact of an arts project is that those who are intended to benefit from the project should decide whether or not they have in fact benefited.

All this affirms for us that medicine is made by and for people. This first section closes with Anne Borsay reminding us that the same is true of history and in particular the history of medicine itself. Identifying medical history as a social practice helps us to make sense of the historical experiences of medicine in their proper context and, of course, to make sense of our own experiences of medicine today. Borsay begins by briefly reviewing the mainstream development of modern European thinking over the past three centuries, noting its reflection in changing conceptions of medical history. She then shows how the changing doctor–patient relationship in this time provides a concrete example of the importance of understanding social and historical context.

The development of this relationship illustrates how emerging medical "cosmologies" are associated with specific political economies and forms of medical knowledge and practice, most notably the bedside model and the hospital model. So, for instance, the bedside model began by emphasising the cataloguing of symptoms and experiences; this rather unscientific "speculative pathology" gave way at the theoretical level to the scientific revolution and an associated transformation in the foundations of medical knowledge. Hospital medicine, judged now against the historical record, proclaims the differentiation of distinct disease entities and relegates symptoms to second place. But Borsay points out that theoretical developments were not necessarily mirrored in practice. Here the historical picture is more complex, revealing social influences such as patronage and the importance of patients' attitudes to pain, which can sometimes appear to us as incomprehensibly stoical and courageous. Isolated reports of "heroic" medical interventions at that time can distract us from the generally conservative and cautious interventions countenanced at the bedside and in hospitals. Nonetheless, Borsay shows, the overall trend was for the patient narrative gradually to disappear in favour of technical investigation, for symptom to give way to disease entity and for treatment to become non-negotiable. In effect, the humanities gradually retreat from medicine during this period.

Despite the scepticism of postmodernists and empiricists, Borsay maintains that medical history as a social practice offers us a number of practical means of learning from the past. She cites the uses of oral histories as directly therapeutic to the patients who supply them and reviews the use of medical records as scientific data. The influence of the past is an educative one but it does not determine what we shall do or say now. Rather we can say that understanding the past deepens our understanding of the present. This is, then, an important role for the medical humanities in action.

# 1

# The nature and role of the medical humanities

David Greaves

The idea that the study of medicine and healthcare requires a broad approach embracing what would now be regarded as both the arts and science began in antiquity and has lost favour only since the ascendancy of biomedical science in the past two centuries. However, since the 1960s the assumptions underlying the authority of modern scientific medicine have themselves begun to be questioned and this has been manifest in a number of different ways, e.g. the emergence of the anti-psychiatry movement which raised questions about the proper boundaries and expertise of medicine; the inability of science and technology to deal effectively with many chronic and disabling conditions, despite escalating levels of public expenditure on healthcare; and an awareness of the personal insensitivity of much of modern medicine and its failure to take account of the patient's perspective.

The response in terms of the education of healthcare professionals has been much slower to develop in Britain than in the United States, where courses in ethics first emerged in the 1960s and in medical humanities in the 1970s. In Britain medical ethics has only recently been accepted as a compulsory element of the core curriculum for medical students and the wider notion of medical humanities has not yet gained recognition. It would therefore seem appropriate to address some very basic questions concerning the nature of medical humanities and its role in medicine and healthcare.

## The nature of medical humanities

The perception since the 1960s of there being a "crisis" in western medicine has led either explicitly or implicitly to a range of different responses, which are underpinned by varying notions of the nature of medicine, and so also of medical humanities.

## Medicine as a science

Viewed from this perspective, what is required is the further and more sophisticated development of science and technology. This is often combined with the claim that the problems identified have been overstated, reinforcing the idea that they are potentially soluble without any fundamental change of course. This, then, is a conservative position which sees a continuing reliance on a largely unchanged biomedical paradigm as all that is required, leaving no role, or at most a marginal one, for subjects which are not scientific.

## Medicine as an art

In an editorial entitled "Why arts courses for medical curricula?", Calman and Downie suggest that medicine is properly understood as an art, which encompasses science and technology.[1] This perspective does not seek to deny the role of science and technology in medicine, but rather to frame it within a wider conception. The mode of the arts is therefore what is ultimately seen to count, rather than that of traditional medical science. Thus the place of science and technology is subordinated to that of the arts and medicine is viewed as having the character of an art.

## Medicine and the arts as a counterbalance to medicine as science

Throughout the 20th century concerns have been expressed that science and technology have been an ever-increasing and overdominant influence on medicine and that what is required is a renewal of interest in the art of medicine as counterbalance to this trend. It is this position which has probably gained most allegiance in recent years in the definition and development of medical humanities, with medical humanities being equated with medical arts as subjects which can appropriately be counterposed to a range of other subjects described under the heading of medical sciences.

Within this general understanding, though, a variety of different approaches have been followed. The first is simply to provide a list of subjects which are commonly understood as falling under the rubric of the "Humanities" and then apply them to medicine.

Though at first this may appear straightforward and uncontentious, it is not so because how the list is derived will depend on assumptions about what properly constitutes the "Humanities", and this is open to a number of different interpretations:

1 Any subject which is not considered a natural science.
2 Any subject which is not considered a natural or a social science.
3 Any subject, or part of a subject, which does not rely on a quantitative methodology, so that the social sciences may be partially included. This produces a list which tends to be more restrictive than in (1), but less restrictive than in (2), although there is still room for considerable differences of view.[2]
4 Subjects concerned with the uniqueness of individuals rather than generalisation.

These different interpretations all rely on an essentially similar approach, which sees medicine as having two separate aspects, those of an art and a science, the main difference between them being where the line that divides them is drawn. They therefore all depend on the idea of there being discrete realms of arts and sciences which are clearly separable, with humanities being regarded as equivalent to arts.

There are two problems with this, however. One is that the medical arts or humanities are regarded as what is left over after the medical sciences have been defined, so that if the medical sciences become revised and redefined so as to be more inclusive, they will gradually expand and take over areas which were previously the territory of the medical humanities. The second difficulty is with the impression that the role of the medical humanities is principally to provide a counterweight to biomedical science, in such a way as to humanise the medical enterprise but without producing any fundamental challenge to it. This is because the traditional separation between the medical sciences and medical humanities is maintained and for this to be overcome, an altogether different and more radical approach is required.

## A different conception of medicine and medical humanities

The central problems associated with the three positions identified so far are that they make either the art of medicine or the science of medicine paramount or, in acknowledging the importance of both, provide a sharp separation between them. A more satisfactory position needs to address both these issues and the final position suggested here attempts to do so.

It involves returning to the meaning of the word humanities, rather than assuming that either the "art of medicine" or "the arts" in relation to medicine are necessarily interchangeable with medical humanities. Engelhardt has suggested that the central goal of the humanities is:

> ... to provide an understanding of the human condition through a disciplined examination of the ideas, values and images that frame the significance of the human world and guide human practices...[3]

What this does is to focus attention on the humanities as providing an understanding of the human condition and the values associated with the word "human". Such values cannot then be restricted to any traditional boundaries of particular subjects or methods and are equally applicable to both arts and science subjects. Newell and Gabrielson express this as follows.

> The key word in the term *human*-ities is "human". The humanities share in common this focus on the human – the human being in the human condition – the cultural and creative expressions, values, outlooks, attitudes and lifestyles of *homo sapiens*. Any discipline which has this focus is a humanities discipline and any time other disciplines focus in this way they are humanistic. Thus archaeology, history, comparative religion, and even the so-called hard sciences are rightfully said to be engaged in humanities pursuits in contexts in which they are able to focus in this way.[4]

So the medical humanities are defined in terms of a humanistic perspective and this embodies a mode of enquiry which is typical of philosophy in particular, but can also be discerned in every subject in its relationship with medicine. For example, in the 1960s, Carr described the need for historians to develop a philosophy of history by which he meant a critically reflective outlook towards taking facts for granted, which he suggests was conspicuously absent in the 19th century.

This was the age of innocence, and historians walked in the Garden of Eden, without a scrap of philosophy to cover them, naked and unashamed before the god of history.

Since then, we have known Sin and experienced a Fall; and those historians who today pretend to dispense with a philosophy of history are merely trying, vainly and self-consciously, like members of a nudist colony, to recreate the Garden of Eden in their garden suburb.[5]

This need for a "philosophical outlook" is now widely recognised as being universally applicable to the sciences as well as the arts. As  an illustration of this, Oliver Sacks" reflections on his practice are notable examples of such an outlook being applied without distinction between art and science, so that his "philosophical" observations about the scientific aspects of neurology form an integral part of his work.[6] Thus any attempt to exclude this component would be not only artificial but fatal to his whole enterprise. What this requires, though, is a distinction between the use of the word "philosophy" in connection with a general approach of relevance to any subject and philosophy as a particular subject. It is the former which is being referred to here.[7]

It is then the desire to foster a humanistic perspective using such a philosophical approach which provides an underlying unity within a great diversity of disciplines. Regarded in this way, the subject of medical humanities has two characteristic features. First, it takes human values, both personal and social, as the focus of interest and as applicable to both the arts and the sciences; and second, it is informed by a method appropriate to all those disciplines which are of relevance to medicine. In fact, these two aspects represent two facets of the same issue. It is the irreducibly human nature of medicine which determines both that no aspect of medicine can be divorced from it and also that a philosophical approach is required if it is to be adequately represented.

A further reason for conceptualising medical humanities in this way is that the overall effect of recognising that a humanistic perspective touches on all subjects as they relate to medicine should be to enhance and enrich the insights which each of them would be able to generate and develop on its own. This is not intended to detract from the fact that each subject has its own unique contribution and that the more varied the disciplines included, the greater the potential insights that may be achieved by virtue of their additive input. Rather it is to acknowledge both the possibility of a potentiating effect and also that the larger the number of subjects involved, the greater the need for a common theme and purpose which transcends the individual subjects and so gives coherence to the notion of medical humanities.

The strengths of this conceptualisation of medical humanities are that it recaptures something of the ancient idea that art and science in medicine are inextricably linked, whilst acknowledging that modern science and technology have become the dominant aspect of contemporary medicine and are of a different kind and order from that of antiquity. Yet it also recognises that however sophisticated and powerful science and technology have become, they remain properly the subject of a wider unifying perspective that is humanistic. Indeed, as Lewis Mumford appreciated, it is only by developing such a perspective that humanity can hope to confront the problems that science and technology pose.

> If we are to save technology itself from the aberrations of its present leaders and putative gods, we must in both our thinking and our action come back to the human center; for it is there that all significant transformations begin and terminate.[8]

What will be required if this is taken on board is a willingness to envisage a medical restructuring of both the art and science of medicine. Indeed, medical humanities cannot be adequately understood within the more traditional framework of medicine as science counterbalanced by the arts.

On consideration of these four approaches to the nature of medicine and of medical humanities, the first two may readily be discarded – those in which either art or science predominates. The other two approaches contrast in several ways and deserve more serious consideration. The first equates medical humanities with the medical arts, as subjects which can both be set against and complement medical sciences and this is probably the view most commonly taken of the nature of medical humanities.

The second approach focuses on the human as relevant to the whole of medicine and so cuts across the traditional formulation of western medicine as comprising separate realms of art and science, with the human aspects restricted mainly, if not exclusively, to the former. Thus it cannot readily be captured within the familiar categories of medical arts and sciences or medicine as art and science.

The contrast between these two views can be brought out by

describing them respectively as referring to *the* "medical humanities", on the one hand, and "medical humanities", on the other. To avoid confusion, though, the former, narrower view might be better called the "medical arts" with the term "medical humanities" being reserved for the latter, more general conception. The "medical arts" are then restricted to an engagement of medicine with the liberal arts, so linking together a range of subjects, variously defined, to match that of medical science. However, this is without any unifying conception, other than the contrast made with science. The principal aim is therefore usually seen as being to provide a "balance" to medical science, rather than having any direct influence on it. "Medical humanities", on the other hand, provides an innovative and unified approach which transcends the present structure of medicine as a divided discipline, so allowing for a reappraisal of medical theory and knowledge whilst at the same time enabling practitioners to develop a more rounded and humane attitude to their practice.

This second view is regarded as preferable for two reasons. First because it challenges the division of medicine into separate realms of art and science, which is at the heart of many of its current difficulties, and thus holds out the prospect of developing new ways of resolving them. Second, because it is compatible with the narrower view of "medical arts", which can be readily subsumed under the wider conception of "medical humanities".

## The role of the medical arts and medical humanities

There are a number of possible reasons for studying and making use of both the medical arts and medical humanities as defined above and some of them will be considered here under three main headings.

### Recreation, relaxation, and therapy

It is often suggested that because the education and training of healthcare professionals is so heavily dominated by medical science and technology, it should be balanced by a degree of exposure to the arts. Some introduction to and familiarity with literature, for example, is then extolled either as a good thing in its own right or for its ability to provide entertainment and relaxation. A further extension of this argument is that because healthcare professionals are placed in situations of exceptional stress, teaching them the arts may prove a helpful strategy in dealing with it. In essence, this is a kind of therapy, which has also been a recent subject of interest for patients, especially the mentally ill.

In all these cases, it is clear that it is the medical arts which are being referred to rather than medical humanities.

## Professional education and development

The same starting point as above may also be used to make a different case: that studying the arts will improve the practice of professionals and the quality of patient care. Again, the emphasis has often been on teaching the medical arts rather than medical humanities. However, some authors take the argument further by stressing that they expect such teaching to have a direct impact on clinical practice. Pellegrino (p.3), for example, makes the point as follows.

> Rarely are the humanities in medicine assessed for what they are – neither educational flourishes nor panaceas but indispensable studies whose everyday use is as important for the quality of clinical decisions as the basic sciences are now presumed to be.[2]

This then suggests an awareness of the need to develop and teach medical humanities rather than just the medical arts.

## The social role of medicine

The reasons for developing and studying the medical arts and medical humanities given above are concerned with the effect of such study on individuals, either professionals or patients or both. There are, however, further reasons relating to the role of medicine as an institution within society and two aspects will be considered here.

First, medicine is necessarily shaped by the society of which it is a part, but it also plays an important role in shaping society's norms and values. Over the past 30 years or so the previously shared consensus about the proper nature and role of western medicine has begun to be questioned and a debate has developed about the whole future of medicine and healthcare. As a central focus has been on the way in which the orthodox medical model has subordinated human values to technology and science (or, more correctly, scientism), the interpretation of the medical humanities which sees them as involving not just the arts but a humanistic perspective is of key importance in taking this debate forward.

This concerns not only the role of human values in medicine but it also reflects wider changes within society and in this context, it may have a very special, even unique role. Renée Fox, who has analysed the modern development of bioethics in the United States, which has emerged in parallel with this debate and as one expression of it, suggests that besides its declared purpose, bioethics also functions as an acceptable focus in which the most significant and profound aspects of people's lives can be brought into the open, in a society which has lost many of the traditional means of exploring them.[9] She is also critical of the way in which bioethics had tended to concentrate on a narrow range of issues and employ a restrictive philosophical method and the more eclectic medical humanities approach should counter this trend and so enrich this process.[10]

# Conclusion

A number of reasons have been considered for developing and promoting the study of the medical arts and medical humanities. Although it is the medical arts which are being referred to in relation to recreation, relaxation and therapy, and medical humanities when considering the wider social role of medicine, there appears to be some uncertainty about which is appropriate in respect of professional education and development and in this instance they are not always clearly distinguished. This may then give the appearance that the medical arts and medical humanities, as earlier defined, are not properly separable but simply two aspects of the same discipline. While they may and often do overlap, the argument that their role and purpose are very different will be maintained.

It is often assumed that if all healthcare professionals received a liberal arts education in addition to their current healthcare training, this would be bound to lead to their becoming more rounded and humane practitioners. However, this is not necessarily the case, because if medical science and technology continue to be perceived as the central focus which remains untouched by the medical arts, the core values and methods of clinical practice will remain largely unchanged. The medical arts may well encourage some practitioners to treat patients as people, in addition to treating their diseases, but will have no impact on the conceptualisation of the latter. For others it may have little or no impact at all, because while the underlying message of the centrality of science remains pre-eminent, other concerns are readily ignored.

In contrast with this, the medical humanities perspective raises deeper questions concerning assumptions which are usually taken for granted and are of relevance to the whole of medicine. Promoting medical humanities, then, requires not just an addition to the curriculum but a permeation and change of orientation of the culture of medicine, which will transform not only clinical practice but also the theoretical basis and social structures of medicine and healthcare. Although formal education has an important part to play in this, unless it becomes part of this much wider process, its influence will be relatively marginal.

Teaching the medical arts is fully compatible with developing medical humanities in this way but their purposes are different. The medical arts are essentially an ornament to medicine, whilst the medical humanities are an integral part of it. The medical arts are aimed at humanising practitioners, medical humanities is aimed at humanising medicine.

## References and notes

1   Calman K, Downie R. Why arts courses for medical curricula? *Lancet* 1996; **347**: 1499–1500.
2   For example, Pellegrino inclines to this view but tends to focus rather narrowly on ethics, philosophy, history, law and theology: Pellegrino ED. *Humanism and the Physician*. Knoxville: University of Tennessee Press, 1979: 4.
3   Engelhardt HT Jnr. *The Foundations of Bioethics*. Oxford: Oxford University Press, 1986: 11.
4   Newell JD, Gabrielson IW (eds). *Medicine Looks at the Humanities*. London: University Press of America, 1987: xvii.
5   Carr EH. *What is History?* Harmondsworth: Penguin,1964: 20.
6   For example Sacks O. *A Leg to Stand On*. London: Picador, 1986.
7   If the terms "philosophy" and "philosophical" used in this way cause confusion they are better dropped. It is the idea being conveyed, rather than the words, which is important.
8   Mumford L. *The Myth of the Machine, the Pentagon of Power*. New York: Harcourt Brace Jovanovich, 1970: 240.
9   Fox R. The evolution of American bioethics. Paper given to the Welsh Section of the British Sociology Association Medical Sociology Group in Swansea on 1 May 1997.
10  In contrast, Kopelman argues that bioethics and humanities have much in common and should be regarded as part of the same general field of study. Kopelman LM. Bioethics and humanities: what makes us one field? *J Med Philosophy* 1998; **23**: 356–68.

# 2

# Society, community, well-being

Ray Pahl

It is now widely accepted that there is a direct link between social support and health. There has been a dramatic increase in the number of articles on this topic in medical journals in recent years and a soundly based body of knowledge has accumulated.[1] In an article in the *Journal of the American Medical Association*, published in 1997, an apparently uncontroversial statement prefaced the detailed reporting of results.[2]

> [T]he relative risk for mortality among those with less diverse networks is comparable in magnitude to the relation between smoking and mortality from all causes... Social networks may play a role in the ability of the host to resist infection.

These are large claims and put a heavy responsibility on social scientists to make their putative contribution to health and well-being as clear and as accessible as possible.

There is undoubtedly a danger that those with a traditional medical education may be suspicious of what may appear to them to be overinflated claims. The technical terms used by sociologists may be dismissed as jargon, without recognising that the medical literature is full of technical terms, which are necessary aids in precise description. Furthermore, the findings of sociologists, however initially counterintuitive they may be, are sometimes dismissed as "obvious", once the connections have been explored and explained. Finally, even if the links between social support and forms of well-being are, in general, understood and accepted, there may still be resistance to accepting the consequences. Whilst it may be acceptable for health professionals to advocate changes in, say, a patient's diet, they may jib at the suggestion that some form of intervention in their pattern of social relationships would also be desirable. Some forms of social engineering are more acceptable than others and, of course, some are easier to achieve. The relation between smoking and mortality is now widely understood: the high rates of taxation on tobacco are socially acceptable, as is the insistence that advertisements should carry health warnings or that tobacco should not be sold to children.

However, it would be quite another matter for the government to set precise guidelines for people to generate diverse social networks for themselves, however desirable that might be for their health and well-being. This might appear to be overintrusive. The same problem affects researchers. Asking precise questions about diet or exercise is now coming to be recognised as legitimate, since these are now widely understood to be related to life-threatening conditions, such as heart disease or cancer. However, asking detailed questions about an individual's pattern of social connectedness can in some ways appear more threatening: it raises more fundamental questions about who one is as a person. Those who overindulge in fatty food, sugar or alcohol may decide to justify it in terms of hedonistic pleasure. However, it is more difficult to justify a lifestyle that is lonely and bereft of friends. Such a person would see himself as a "faulty interactant", in Goffman's phrase. Indeed, much of Goffman's work is concerned to demonstrate the various styles of impression management and ways of presenting ourselves that we adopt to maintain socially acceptable identities.[3] We are all, in some sense, what others let us be.

It is a commonplace of sociology to recognise that there are fundamental societal determinants of health and it matters a great deal whether we were born in St Petersburg or St Albans when considering mortality rates. But there are also substantial variations within societies, socially as well as geographically. Finally, within specific locales there are structured variations in social support.

In a review published in the *Lancet*, the authors remark: For all the excitement caused by the new genetics and concern over pollution and emergence of new infections, social variables remain the most important determinants of health. The central importance of poverty and inequality has been well rehearsed in a number of national and international official reports over the last 20 years and I do not propose to elaborate on these here.[4] Similarly, the significance of social class has been well documented, most thoroughly, perhaps, in the longitudinal study of civil servants in Britain – the so-called Whitehall Study.[5]

Without wishing to minimise in any way the importance of those macro-structures in the determination of well-being, I intend to focus in the rest of this chapter on the micro-social worlds in which people generate and maintain their significant sets of social relationships. Unreflectively one might leap to the false conclusion that this was another way of referring to the familiar topics of undergraduate courses in sociology, namely family and community. For a number of reasons I would prefer to avoid slipping too readily into such an assumption.

Let us begin by considering the notion of community, often held to be an unqualified "good thing", rather like parks and motherhood. However, it is evident that strong communities very often arose out of isolation, deprivation or a common external threat. The strength of occupational communities, based on docks, steel mills or mines, may have had strong male solidarities but these were likely to be focused on beer, tobacco, and fatty foods. Whilst these, in the past, may have provided comfort in the context of isolation and material deprivation, few would urge a return to such traditional communities. When the economic base of these solidaristic communities collapsed, so also did the basis for social support: indeed, the very traditions and customs that helped to make the previous exploitation and gender inequalities bearable generally inhibited change and the grasping of new opportunities. Often traditional communities became polarised when newcomers arrived, either as commuters or as workers with different skills in newly established industries. Rivalries, feuds, animosities and the emergence of new divisions have been well documented in a collection of "community studies" carried out in Britain from the 1930s to the 1970s.

The recognition of the "myth of community studies" or the "eclipse of community", to take two titles from the period of disillusion in the 1960s and 1970s, led to a refocus on the idea of social network, which has come in recent years to be a kind of fashionable substitute for the discredited notion of community. Research became more ego centred: that is to say, all the social linkages based on a given individual were mapped, together with the interconnections, if any, between them. This was a very time-consuming exercise but it did allow for quite a high degree of mathematical sophistication based on graph theory. Networks were analysed in terms of both morphological and interactional characteristics: the former were anchorage, density, reachability, and range; the latter were content, directedness, durability and intensity. When these ideas were first discussed in the late 1960s, mainly by social anthropologists many of whom had done fieldwork in Central Africa, considerable intellectual excitement was generated. There were high hopes of a dramatic and disciplined advance in the theoretical understanding of social relations and social connectedness.

For a number of reasons this promise was not realised. Anthropologists could manage to study social networks in certain kinds of locales and they certainly did extend their ethnography to describe merchant bankers or the links between financial and corporate elites in the City of London. However, such was the effort involved in gaining the complex social information that, after a time, it seemed that the means of analysing and conceptualising the data became the very ends of the research itself. Furthermore, the complexities of handling detailed social network data as it contracted or expanded over time overwhelmed most researchers.

Not surprisingly, perhaps, those who were concerned with practical policy questions, notably academic social gerontologists, whilst continuing to use the term "social network", operationalised it in a more limited and manageable way. They were concerned with describing what I prefer to call personal communities: that is, the number of people who are socially significant to an individual based on a number of functional and emotional criteria. Such people could be described as friends, acquaintances, family members, neighbours or whatever.

Before continuing further, I want to put forward similar qualification and doubts in relation to the term "family". Empirical research has shown that sets of roles, duties, and responsibilities cannot be, as it were, read off from different kinds of agnatic or affinal ties. Increasingly, it has been shown that people may be more or less close to parents, siblings and so forth depending on how well they "get on". Social and geographical mobility helps to weaken some ties and to strengthen others. Mothers who expect daughters to follow traditional paths may be disturbed or estranged from them by alternative feminist values or sexual and gender identities. Sibling rivalries can be avoided by maintaining social or geographical distance. As rates of divorce and separation increased with concomitant growth of stepfamilies, the notion of "stable family life" appeared elusive and ambiguous. Politicians, somewhat desperately seeking to support what they perceived to be a form of social glue essential to the maintenance of social cohesion, found themselves endlessly urging the shutting of the stable door after the horse had bolted.

This is in no way to suggest that most people do not recognise, support, and aspire to the idea that dependent children need loving parents. However, the period of parenting is a relatively short part of an extended life course and "the family" includes many sets and types of relationships. The daughter aged two is unlikely to be that different now from her grandmother at that age. However, the daughter aged 22 or 52 is likely to be very different. Few would now be prepared or be expected to give up marriage or a career in order to care for an elderly parent. These arguments are very familiar and do not need to be elaborated further. Without necessarily adopting the phrase "families or choice", which originated in the gay community, it is nevertheless true that the meaning and significance of kin links have to be discovered, not assumed.

As long ago as 1978 Mark Abrams conducted a survey for Age Concern in which he found that good friends and neighbours were considered more important than family for a satisfying life. Later, in 1987 Peter Willmott carried out research for the Policy Studies Institute in London and in his report *Friendship Networks and Social Support* demonstrated the complexities of social support. Friends were the main confidantes for those sharing personal problems. Willmott also noted that "there was nothing which was wholly the preserve of relatives or friends".

In the light of this and other survey evidence, it is plausible to suggest that friends are becoming more kin-like in their capacity to provide a variety of forms of social support and kin are becoming more friend-like, as people choose which members of their family they want to involve more closely in their lives. Empirical research on friends and friendship at the University of Essex has just been completed and the first wave of interviews has already provided some support for this cross-suffusion theory.

We are attempting to map people's personal communities and the way we do this is as follows. First we provide respondents with 20 adhesive labels and ask them to write on each those people who are most important to them in their lives now. These can be family, friends, neighbours, work colleagues or whatever and they are not obliged to use all 20 labels. Then, at the time of the interview we bring a chart of five concentric circles and ask respondents to stick each label on the chart in order of most importance or closeness, with the inner circle representing the sphere of greatest closeness with the respondent being in the middle point. They can use as many of the concentric circles as they consider appropriate.

As one might expect, family members tend to dominate in the innermost circle but interestingly this is not always so. There is an understandable hesitancy in putting parents further out but some respondents, somewhat apologetically to be sure, put one or both of their parents in a more distant ring. Siblings can be in any of the five rings. By talking through the placement of the labels with the interviewer, respondents work out, perhaps for the first time, who really counts in their lives and why. Of course, their personal communities have to be analysed in terms of gender, age, class and much else besides before any kind of pattern or generalisation can be discerned or made. However, it is absolutely certain that we shall be able to document a very substantial diversity in people's personal communities.

In very brief outline, I am arguing first, that the notions of family and community are too ambiguous, imprecise and contested to serve as a basis for an understanding of social support. Second, the term "social network" has been used too loosely, the complexities of analysis have become ends in themselves and the actual qualitative content of the links that are charted are more often assumed than seriously explored. I suggest that the term "personal community", being the actual set of social relationships that is significant for an individual at a particular point in time, is in fact relatively easy to define very precisely and, most importantly, can be explored qualitatively to reveal meanings and significances.

However, snapshots are not enough. There is an urgent need to see how personal communities change over time as people go through vicissitudes of the life course. The personal community of a student at college will be different from that when she is a young mother or when she has returned to employment. Personal communities in retirement will be different again. Of course, some friends from childhood may provide support throughout the life course, as may siblings. The term "social convoy" has been used to describe the changing pattern of personal communities as one goes through the life course. It might sometimes be appropriate to refer to such a social convoy as a social network: this would be the case, for example, if someone stayed in the same geographical area, so that throughout life the personal community remained largely composed of family or school friends who had also stayed in the same area. There may then be an almost complete overlap between all the members of people's personal communities and their social convoys, thus providing a distinctive locality-based social network. Such may be the case in long-established farming areas but it is likely to be relatively rare in modern Britain. It is more likely that people will have moved away for education, employment, marriage, remarriage, more employment changes and on retirement. Individual members of the social convoy will be added from different contexts or at different stages of the life course but it is very unlikely that they will know each other. Small clusters of fellow students or neighbours will make up mini-networks but as life goes on some will fall by the wayside.

It is clear that we have to be wary about all-encompassing terms such as social support or the currently very fashionable notion of social capital and their connection with health and well-being. We have to explore precisely which kinds of social connectedness, encompassing which kinds of qualitative needs and functions relate to which kinds of health outcomes. Furthermore, correlation does not imply causation and there needs to be a much greater focus on processes. It may well be that some of the results which link social support to better health and well-being could be obtained by substituting the ownership of cats or dogs for social support.

The Health Education Authority, before being closed down, established a programme of studies based on the notion of social capital, in the hope that theoretical models could be developed which might enable research findings to be linked with policy and practice. The idea would be to devise "social capital" indicators to put alongside the other factors affecting health, such as the quality of the physical environment, housing or transport.

In the report *Social Capital and Health*, Catherine Campbell and colleagues conducted a most interesting study of two wards in Luton. One, Farley, had lower levels of health quality than Sundon Park and the researchers attempted to discover whether there were substantial differences in the sense of local identity, trust, reciprocal help and support, and civic engagement between the two areas. In the event, certain interesting social differences between the two areas did indeed emerge. However, the researchers found that certain dimensions of social capital were more relevant to health than others. Community identity seemed less important, whereas trust and civic engagement were more salient. They concluded: "More attention needs to be paid to the small-scale, *informal networks of friends and neighbours* which formed the bulk of the social capital available to informants in both our wards" (my emphasis). There was a modest degree of small-scale community activism and this also varied between the high-health and the low-health wards. This was essentially an exploratory study and was acknowledged to be aiming to do no more than open up promising directions for future research. The authors use the word "community" simply to refer to a particular locale: they do not let the word carry normative assumptions about what constitutes a "good" community.

This is just as well. Some of the powerfully interconnected "communities" can be very inward-looking and bound together by norms and values at variance, if not in conflict, with those of the host society. Certain criminal gangs can induce considerable social cohesion amongst their members. Similarly, immigrant communities gain a sense of identity and continuity with their previous homeland by keeping apart from the host society.

The authors of the HEA study mentioned above rightly recognise that once a precise understanding of social support and social networks – or what I prefer to call personal communities – is reached, the problem of how "better" personal communities can be promoted becomes pertinent. This raises tricky ethical questions of social engineering and before coming to my own suggestions, I want to provide an illustration of the difficulties.

In a recent piece of empirical sociological research carried out in the United States, Rebecca Adams and Rosemary Blieszner attempted to discover whether those structurally advantaged early in life were better placed to have good, supportive friends in old age. Not unreasonably, it might be assumed that those more financially secure, with higher levels of education, would have more means and opportunities to acquire and retain friends. Those rich in cultural capital are more likely to accumulate social capital, as the current jargon has it. Those assessing elderly people and perceiving the signs of cultural capital – books, CDs, etc. – in the home and meeting an articulate, well-educated person might well imagine that these are valid indications that such a person would be less likely to need public support. Furthermore, if such people were found to have problematic friendships – being too close or demanding or just fading away – such friendships could be readily replaced by their superior social skills and networking capacities.

The study was carried out in Greensboro, North Carolina in 1990 and was based on 28 women and 25 men aged between 55 and 84 years. These respondents acknowledged various degrees of "problematic" friendships, since half of them mentioned a friendship that was "difficult" and two-thirds reported a friendship that was "fading away".

Much to the researchers' surprise, the results of their study were directly counter to their initial expectations. Problematic friendships were actually more likely amongst the "young-old", financially better-off women or those in the upper-middle class. These are the very people that, on the face of it, one would expect to be securely socially bonded. Women are conventionally perceived to be better "friend-makers" and *a fortiori* this would apply to those in the more financially secure upper-middle class.

Once the researchers had their counterintuitive results, they were obliged to devise some new hypotheses. Maybe those who have always been able to make friends easily were more able to dump problematic friends, believing that they would be easily replaced. Perhaps the culturally advantaged have higher expectations of friendship and because of the strength of their own resources, they have preferred to let old friends fade away, rather than get entangled in emotionally exhausting relationship work. Such a cynical supposition would suggest that perhaps the structurally privileged elderly in Greensboro are not particularly amiable people. Alternatively, the authors suggest, the friend-dumpers may just be more honest and confident and the lower-middle class respondents were, in colloquial terms, more mealy mouthed. The authors recognise that their research may create ethical difficulties for those concerned with social policy or what they call "individual or group intervention [i.e. social engineering] aimed at both those with few friends and those with problematic relationships".

In some ways this is rather an alarming study, especially if it is symptomatic of an emerging managerial social science which is too eager to move on from attempting to understand what is, to prescribing what ought to be. Even if social scientists agree with their colleagues in private that they hold to the spirit of Max Weber's discussion of values and objectivity, they may still collude with professional social fixers, if only to ensure funding for their research. The authors, to my astonishment, suggest two possibly useful programmes arising out of their research. The first programme would be designed "to help structurally disadvantaged people articulate problems in their relationships [i.e. stop the poor and insecure being so mealy mouthed] and create opportunities for finding new friends" [i.e. go out and smile to get someone to do your shopping for you]. The second programme would be to help the structurally-advantaged people "to make decisions regarding the acquisition, repair and termination of friends" [i.e. don't dump your friends dear, you never know when you may need them].

Unfortunately, it is easy to mock so much of the over-earnest research on friendship and it may be hard on these two particular researchers who are among the most respected in the field. In fairness to them, they do conclude by recognising that having more friends does not necessarily imply that an elderly person receives more social support. It may equally imply that such a person has more worries and relationship problems.

At the risk of short-cutting a long and complex argument, let me say categorically that certain kinds of personal communities help to keep people happier and healthier and to live longer. Some of the best and most robust evidence relates to careful longitudinal studies of men and women suffering from coronary heart disease. Those with better emotional support are much more likely to recover and to live longer. In one study among those admitted to hospital after heart attack, almost 38% of those who reported no source of emotional support died in the hospital compared with 11.5% of those with two or more sources of support. Living alone is also an independent risk factor.

So what to do? It is clear that what is important is not simply the quantity but also, crucially, the quality of social connectedness and many would argue that some people are simply less good at forming close and supportive friendships. Some developmental psychologists can appear highly deterministic by suggesting that patterns of attachment to a mother or mother substitute in infancy can have direct consequences for patterns of social attachment later in life. This brings us back to the "faulty interactant" argument mentioned above.

The idea that suitable friends can be provided for the "friend challenged" is clearly ludicrous. The kind of friend that is most needed is the one who can make the subject feel cared for and loved and to believe that he or she is esteemed and valued. Furthermore, it is also advantageous if the subject belongs to a network of communication and mutual obligation. It is very unlikely that such social support can be easily provided institutionally, however essential it may be to health and well-being.

The best hope, in my judgement, is to encourage ways in which people can join in common activities together. Often well-meaning people provide activities in "community centres" which are not well attended or not appropriate for those most in need. Clearly the arts could play a central role here, not in providing spectacles but in engaging people in common activities. Of course, a considerable amount of such activity goes on but it is not, perhaps, given the serious support it deserves. I am thinking of the various projects in rural areas by the Women's Institutes to gather information about times past, whether in the form of photographs and other objects or in memories and reminiscences. This kind of work is immensely important and gives many elderly people, perhaps in hospital or residential homes, a strong sense of being esteemed and valued. Those who feel they have lived a rather ordinary and humble life can be greatly invigorated and encouraged by the interest taken by oral or local historians in their memories of everyday experiences.

Of course, local history is not limited to the countryside and this is but one example of a host of activities that could involve people. Facilitators and enablers in a variety of projects throughout the country know that social contacts are made in the cracks. People get to know each other when the caretaker doesn't turn up in time and they have to make conversation as they are waiting to enter the hall.

This line of thinking is not novel: personal communities grow and develop from common engagement in activities. This has been well theorised by George Homans in his classic work *Social Behaviour: its Elementary Forms*. It also does not need emphasising that there are many trends in society that prevent people from engaging in these life-enhancing activities.

The report to the Nuffield Trust *A User's Guide to the Practice and Benefits of Arts in Healthcare and Healthy Living* is a useful compendium of activities and practices, but it does not tell us how these activities might produce appropriate sentiments and social support. Much more needs to be known about the meaning and nature of the actual social interactions that take place when people gather together for different purposes. In some cases the gathering together might actually reduce people's self-esteem if the atmosphere appears competitive or if new social anxieties are generated. For example, people from a variety of social backgrounds may gather together to take part in choral singing. The activity takes up all the available time while they are together and people leave quickly at the end to catch buses or to drive home. A well-meaning social secretary may then devise different occasions at which people "may get to know each other". This might involve, say, a buffet supper in which people find themselves obliged to mix together at tables sitting six or eight people. The social equality based on similar singing capacity may then be undermined by an awareness of social and economic distinctions. Variations in social and cultural capital may then serve to create embarrassment and anxiety. This may seem overly pessimistic: new friendships may be created which may blossom in all kind of ways. However, evidently, there is friendship and friendship. The health-supporting type of friendship is of a different order from the superficial acquaintance or what Aristotle referred to as the friends of pleasure.

I recognise that I am introducing complexities and ambiguities at the point in this chapter when I should, perhaps, be offering some encouraging conclusions. This is inevitable, given that I have not completed the analysis of the research I mentioned above and I am understandably cautious in forecasting its results. However, one thing is clear: the enormous variety of people's personal communities which can be categorised in many different ways suggests that there can be no easy social "fix" arising from greater understanding. Friendship is also a highly complex social process and is related to variations based on, for example, gender, age and social context more generally. Curiously, however, the subject has received only modest scholarly attention and its significance for health and well-being has been recognised only very recently.

Those who are engaged in medical research may raise an eyebrow at the idea that research on friends and friendship can have practical importance in their field. However, a number of technical papers have now rigorously established the correlation between social connectedness and social, psychological and physical well-being.[6] The task that must now be addressed is to open up the black box of social causation. Simply listing various worthy cultural and artistic activities in a locality and then assuming that this is an indication of enhanced well-being will not do. If one consequence could be the drawing apart of those with greater cultural capital from those with lesser, then the consequences for the less privileged may be negative. This, of course, is not an original insight: there has been much speculation on such issues.[7]

However, I hope that I have said enough to suggest that far from being a marginal or self-indulgent research topic, the nature, range, functions and meaning of forms of friendship is an important field to explore. Styles and contexts of friendship are changing in the contemporary world. Surveys show that among young people in western Europe aged between 16 and 34, work or a career is not considered to be "really important to them personally". Of greatest importance to this age cohort was "having friends" (95%) or having enough free time (80%). Only 9% cited work as "the main factor for success in life". Of course, one would want to analyse such survey findings rather carefully. However, there is now a substantial body of evidence to suggest that friends are becoming increasingly salient in the lives of those under 40 and this is likely to carry on through the life course.[8] If a friendly society is also a more healthy society, this trend should be welcomed. Likewise those tendencies in contemporary society that may inhibit or reduce the emergence of friend-like relationships need to be analysed and possibly, if appropriate, inhibited or restrained.

# References and notes

1   For recent and useful reviews of this topic see Cohen S. Psychosocial models of the role of social support in the etiology of physical disease. *Health Psychol* 1988; 7: 269–97. Uchino BA *et al*. The relationship between social support and physiological processes: a review with emphasis on underlying mechanisms and implications for health. *Psychol Bull* 1996; **119**: 488–531. Elstad JI. The psychosocial perspective in social inequalities in health. *Sociol Illness Health* 1998; **20**: 698–718.

2   Cohen S. Social ties and susceptibility to the common cold. *JAMA* 1997; **277**: 1940–1.

3   See, for example, Goffman E. *The Presentation of Self in Everyday Life*. New York: Doubleday Anchor Books, 1959, and *Relations in Public*. Harmondsworth: Allen Lane, Penguin Press, 1971.

4   The best place to start would probably be Wilkinson RG. *Unhealthy Societies*. London: Routledge, 1996 or Drever F, Whitehead M, *Health Inequalities*. London: Office for National Statistics, 1997. Wilkinson has stimulated a most useful debate. Something of the flavour of this can be found in Muntaner C *et al*. The social class determinants of income inequalities and social cohesion. *Int J Health Services* 1999; **29**: 699–732.

5   The results of this longitudinal study have been published in a variety of academic journals. See, for example, Rael EGS *et al*. Sickness absence in the Whitehall II study, London: the role of social support and material problems. *J Epidemiol Comm Health* 1995; **49**:474–81, and Marmot MG *et al*. Health inequalities among British civil servants: the Whitehall II study. *Lancet* 1991; **337**:1387–93.

6   Perhaps the best book with which to get an overall perspective on the field is the collection edited by Sarason BR *et al*. *Social Support: an interactional view*. Chichester: John Wiley, 1990.

7   Two excellent introductions to the idea and significance of social capital are Portes A. Social capital: its origins and applications in modern sociology. *Ann Rev Sociol* 1998; **24**:1–24 and Hall PA. Social capital in Britain. *Br J Political Sci* 1999; **29**:417–61.

8   The research on friendship mentioned in this essay at the University of Essex is entitled *Rethinking Friendship*, ESRC Project R000237836 directed by RE Pahl and E Spencer. An accessible introduction to the literature is Pahl R. *On Friendship*. Cambridge: Polity Press, 2000. See also the chapters by Graham Allan and Kaeren Harrison in Adams RG, Allan G. *Placing Friendship in Context*. Cambridge: Cambridge University Press, 1998.

# 3

# "No appealing solution": evaluating the outcomes of arts and health initiatives

François Matarasso

## "We're not talking about happiness"

At the climax of a recent novel by Bernhard Schlink, a young German law student is faced by a former lover, accused of war crimes in a case he is studying, across a courtroom. He knows something about her which, if it would not render her innocent, would go far towards exonerating her but he also knows that she does not want him to reveal it. She is prepared to be convicted of murder to avoid this being known. One evening, in a turmoil of indecision, he discusses his ethical dilemma with his father who, by the good fortune permitted to novelists, is a professor of philosophy. The answer is unequivocal: the professor acknowledges that the position of children has been neglected by philosophers, but concludes that "With adults I unfortunately see no justification for setting other people's views of what is good for them above their own ideas of what is good for themselves."[1] This is a hard pill for his son to swallow and he asks:

> "Not even if they themselves would be happy about it later?"
> He shook his head. "We're not talking about happiness, we're talking about dignity and freedom. Even as a little boy, you knew the difference. It was no comfort to you that your mother was always right."

As an outsider to both medicine and philosophy this seems to me to be the central issue which we have to address when evaluating the outcomes of any rapprochement between medicine and the humanities. What is good for people and how do we know? If we accept that we are not entitled to impose our view of what is good for someone upon them – albeit with some exceptions such as that highlighted by the recent judgement in favour of a health authority wanting to give a 15 year old a heart transplant against her wishes – what implications does this have for the evaluation, indeed the conduct, of arts and health initiatives?

## Definitions and ambiguities

### Defining art

The sensible place to start trying to elucidate these questions is by clarifying what it is we are talking about. This chapter will refer to the arts rather than using the broader term "humanities" for the sake of a clearer, if more limited focus. One of the problems which British and much western policy has with art is that it tends to mistake the external form signifying an artistic process for the substance of art itself. Thus art is often thought of as a product – a painting, sculpture or performance – which can be recognised and categorised. It is this concept which underpins arguments about whether a poem by Keats is or is not "better" than a song by Bob Dylan. In my view, it leads ultimately to sterile debates which actively exclude most people from participation in the fundamental processes of the arts.

An alternative and more useful way of thinking about art is to focus on the process involved rather than the product.

*Conceptual art — meh.*

Art may be defined as a means through which we can examine our experience of ourselves, the world around us, and the relationship between the two, and share the results with other people in a form which gives free rein to our intellectual, physical, emotional and spiritual qualities.[2]

This conception of art identifies it as one of the tools which humanity has developed for meeting its needs; its essential value is that it permits us to do things which we can do in no other way. Thus art is an exact parallel to science as a human asset. Science, according to Richard Feynman, is a "method of finding things out"[3] and we do not confuse that method, which is an unqualified good since it gives us abilities we would not otherwise have, with its consequences, which may be seen as good, bad or both by different people and societies.

*No!*

Art, then, is a method of exploration and expression. It may be undertaken with more or less integrity and with more or less ability, technique or originality, but the poetry of a mental health service user and the poet laureate use the same method. Its wider value will vary; the work of some artists can resonate for millions of people across time and space, while that of others will be important only to family, friends or even just themselves. They are nonetheless part of the same process. This is a more helpful conception of art because it enables us to understand better what role it plays, or might play, in our lives, whether as makers of art or as its active interpreters. We should think of audiences as actively engaged with the products of artistic processes since the acts of seeing, listening, touching or reading involve a dialogue of sensibility with the artist. And one of the roles of art, we are increasingly coming to appreciate, is to contribute to our well-being, even to our health.

## Not defining health

It is evident that there are at least as many ways of thinking about and defining health as the arts and that our language and concepts for doing so continue to change all the time. Fundamental divisions exist between those who see a norm of good health as under attack from specific malfunctions and those who see health as a fluctuating experience where cause and effect may be highly complex. Over time, we have recognised conditions such as melancholia which have subsequently fallen out of fashion and come to understand new pathologies such as posttraumatic stress disorder. And if that were not enough, we have complicated everything with moral values and judgements which have brought us the "gay plague" and the increasing opprobrium (not to say healthcare restriction) to which smokers are subjected.

These different conceptions produce very different approaches to evaluating health status whose range is illustrated by two contrasting health indices. The Barthel Index was developed in the United States[4] and designed to enable health professionals to assess levels of disability according to a consistent scale; its indicators include "feeding, personal toilet (wash face, comb hair, shave, clean teeth), ascend and descend stairs and controlling bowels". The effect, it must be said, is to see the person as a kind of machine whose performance can be measured and accorded an aggregate value. The Nottingham Health Profile[5] was developed by and with disabled people in response to such dehumanising analyses. It concentrates much more on the individual's experience of disability and its indicators could not be more different: "I'm tired all the time; I find it hard to bend; Everything is an effort; I feel lonely".

Clearly, it would be fruitless to try to define health here but perhaps that is the point: a general definition of good health is impossible since health is always experienced and the value each of us sets on different aspects will vary. Crudely, a musician might be expected to suffer much more from deafness than an accountant. If health is an experience rather than a definable condition, then we can see that it may have a close relationship to art conceived as a method for understanding and expressing experience.

## Some practice

The way into thinking about the relationship between art and health was probably paved in the fields of psychology and psychiatry, where the causes of ill health have always been least open to description through the mechanistic metaphor. Imaginative doctors have encouraged patients with mental health problems to explore their feelings for many years, though with very mixed motives and results. However, although our understanding of the process is little better than the rest of our knowledge of the mind and its effects, it is evident that the arts can have a directly therapeutic value for some patients.

Such experiences may have nurtured the growing interest in the relationship between our health and our minds and, by extension, the arts. We know that the arts cannot mend a broken leg but perhaps they can help a person whose leg is broken by improving the experience of life with a broken leg and consequently its healing. We know that art cannot restore damaged arteries but it may have a role in helping a person with damaged arteries to understand how their lifestyle may be affecting their health and give them greater power to do something about it. Indeed, one of the difficulties which the arts face in relating to medicine and other areas of social policy is that their connection with experience means that they can be shown to have an impact on almost every aspect of life. This has contributed to a lack of focus about what the arts can do and a degree of overclaiming.

### Playing by the right rules

The very term "arts and health" covers a huge range of ideologies, values and practice. In the continuing absence of a proper taxonomy, it is worth clarifying some of this. The critical division is between arts projects, which have health outcomes, and health projects, which use arts methods and may result in arts outcomes.[6]

Activities can have only one aim, though they will usually have many and diverse outcomes. Trying to run a programme with two or more aims is a short route to failure since the aims will sooner or later present conflicting choices arising from the underlying values they embody. Take, for example, the case of a theatre project in a day-care centre: the artistic goal of producing a performance may conflict directly with what is seen to be positive in health terms for the participants. It is possible to run a theatre project with mental health service users with therapeutic outcomes; it is also possible to offer a therapeutic course using theatre. But theatre goals and therapeutic goals cannot be given equal priority because they use different rules. Theatre, for example, cannot exist without degrees of manipulation whose legitimacy we accept when we take part in workshops or as members of an audience: we expect to be deceived, to have our emotional responses played about with, within the limits of theatre. But therapeutic practice is fundamentally opposed to the idea of manipulating or deceiving an individual in order to produce a desired effect. Confusion over the purpose of a project will inevitably result in a clash between competing sets of rules.

This situation may be changing as practice in the field develops. It is possible that a new approach with a single, combined goal drawing on arts and health objectives is emerging, but there is neither sufficient evidence nor understanding to be sure. At present, it is probably wiser to accept that projects will fall into one type or the other and that those which do not are more likely to be confused about their values and purpose than to be forging a new type of practice.

## Types of practice

Within that overall division, there are currently many different ways in which the arts are making a contribution to health promotion, of which the most significant may be briefly noted. Each strand, it scarcely needs to be said, embraces a very broad range of practice and values.

- Art therapy and rehabilitation through arts workshops.
- Environmental arts programmes designed to improve the

appearance or atmosphere of health facilities.
- Performances within health and social care institutions.
- Health education initiatives through presentation of information through media such as theatre, video, CD-ROM or through direct participation in workshops.
- Art workshops for patients, medical staff or both together where the purpose is cultural and social rather than expressly therapeutic.
- The use of the arts in training and support of medical professionals.

There are a number of characteristics that distinguish between these types of initiative, not least the extent of their ambitions, but in terms of how we might approach their evaluation, the most important difference is probably the degree to which decision making is shared among all those involved. At one extreme, control may reside in a single person – hospital administrator, consultant, artist – at the other it may be a genuinely collaborative process involving all those with an interest in a project. It is the initiatives tending towards the latter end of the spectrum that are of most interest in the present discussion.

# The challenge of evaluation

## A grey area

There is a growing body of evidence that the arts have a valuable and wider contribution to make to the fields of medicine and healthcare.[7] However, much work remains to be done in developing understanding of how and why such connections bring benefits and in developing consistent practice in their exploitation.

But these benefits also present big challenges for policy and planning of health services because they are so indistinct. They relate very often to how people feel and while there may be measurable reductions in various health problems, it can be difficult to establish causal links between the arts intervention and the outcome.[8] A modern health service, with far more demands than resources, will seek to invest in treatments and procedures that can be shown to bring positive results. It is therefore constantly engaged in complicated assessments of need, cost, likelihood of success and eventual value. New and emerging approaches to healthcare stand little chance of widespread acceptance unless they can demonstrate their cost-effectiveness within this framework.

Those working in the broad area of arts and health therefore face a complicated situation. Most of the benefits resulting from their work are rooted in the experience of health rather than in a scientifically observable and measurable change in pathology; indeed that is their distinctive and additional value in a healthcare programme. But, given the subjective nature of experience, how can systems of evaluation be developed which can do justice to these new approaches while at the same time being credible within the context of dominant medical understanding?

## Distinguishing between impact and value

The first problem in thinking about evaluation is the word itself. We tend to use it to imply a process of careful weighing of evidence in order to determine the truth about an activity or situation. But that is something of a fiction, designed to protect us from having to face up to the fact that evaluation requires us to make judgements based on our values. We behave as if the outcome of an activity, where it can be reliably demonstrated, were equivalent to its value: it is not. The value of a given good (always assuming the outcomes of an activity are goods) is always relative because its purchase necessarily implies another good foregone. Evaluation, properly understood, means assigning a value to something and value is debatable, contestable, political. In healthcare, as in most of public policy, there is a strong reluctance to appear to be making value judgements, though in reality it is done all the time. We need a clearer understanding of the process of evaluation and we need a better vocabulary.

We could instead think of evaluation of public policy and programmes as having two distinct stages. The first, which might be termed "impact assessment", would involve gathering information of kinds and in ways which I shall address shortly. The second would be the process of agreeing what value any identified impact should be assigned and it would involve a much wider constituency, up to and including the general public. This approach would therefore make a clear distinction between the outcomes of an activity and its value. For example, it might be that the demonstrable outcomes of an arts initiative in a maternity hospital include personal benefits for patients, relatives and staff, environmental benefits, healthcare benefits arising from shorter inpatient stays, development of professional skills and practice and artistic benefits. The value of the investment that produced those results would have to be judged by the hospital or other investor against the alternative goods which it might have bought.

Outcomes themselves are relative to inputs and outputs: clearly, effective use of our resources implies securing the best possible ratio between inputs, outputs, and outcomes; we want the most benefit for the least cost (and not just financial cost, as we shall see). So an assessment must identify more than just the outcomes of an activity. Done thoroughly, an impact assessment would describe:

- the original stated aim and objectives of an initiative (this is rarely done well in the arts, but without such a preliminary statement it is almost impossible to demonstrate cause and effect or produce credible evidence of impact)
- the methods planned and used to meet those objectives
- the inputs – staff, money, other resources – required to deliver the methods
- the outputs, in terms of new activity or goods, produced by the inputs
- the outcomes, desired, intended, foreseen or not, resulting from the outputs.

An assessment process which reported this information would provide a solid foundation for an informed discussion about the value of a given initiative.

## Who defines success?

If this approach to evaluation is to be adopted, it is clear that the starting point of any project must be clarification of what it is intended to achieve. And if it is right that each of us is responsible for judging what is best for us, this begs several questions. Who decides what the problem is? Who decides how it should be tackled? And, crucially, who defines the standard of success? In trying to answer these questions, I have proposed six principles which I believe should underpin not just the evaluation of arts projects which have social objectives, but their conduct as a whole.

- Projects intended to produce social benefits should address stated needs or aspirations.

- It is unethical to seek to produce change without the informed consent of those involved.
- The needs and aspirations of individuals or communities are best identified by them, often in partnership with others, such as local authorities, public agencies and arts bodies.
- Partnership requires the agreement of common objectives and commitments (though not all goals need be shared by all partners).
- Those who have identified a goal are best placed to ascertain when it has been met.
- An arts project may not be the most appropriate means of achieving a given goal.[9]

Like all principles, these are aspirational in the sense that it may not be possible to meet all of them in each case. For example, they raise questions about what is meant by informed consent, particularly when people may not be able fully to envisage, for reasons of experience, age or disability, the range of alternatives between which they are asked to choose. That need not be an obstacle to their use, since life is always lived in circumstances less tidy than the way we might wish or talk about it, and for good reason too; what matters is that we have a clear guide for our actions.

## Costs and negative impacts

The second principle reflects the reality that we must individually pay whatever costs ensue from our involvement in the humanities. My concern here is not with the problems caused by poorly executed projects, though they are real, but with the fact that positive outcomes can bring their own costs and difficulties. Change implies growth and with growth come growing pains. One of the most serious issues is that people may see themselves and their relationships differently – something which may or may not be welcomed by others. An experienced community arts worker, Gerri Moriarty, has illustrated some of the problems:

In the mid-Seventies, the project for which I was working ran a small creative writing group, which was mostly attended by young women. At the end of the first year, I was surprised to notice that at least 50% of the group had either separated from their husbands/partners during that period or were considering doing so. It took me a little while to understand that if women

are working regularly in a context that is challenging and affirming, they may not confine their increased self-confidence and
self-esteem to three hours on a Wednesday afternoon.[10]

Is this tally of broken relationships a sign of the positive benefits of
the writing group on the self-confidence of its members? Does it
illustrate the damaging social influence of such activities? Or are we
confronting the complex, difficult and contingent realities of life?
Surely, everything depends on our perspective, political beliefs,
values and personal situation. Such outcomes not only present
ethical and methodological problems to evaluators but also raise
fundamental questions about what is, and what is not, legitimate
practice not just in the humanities or in medicine but in initiatives
which seek to link them. This underlines the importance of
recognising the fundamental philosophical truth that each of us
must judge what is or is not good for us; in this context, that means
being able to choose the nature and extent of our engagement with
the humanities as much as with medicine.

# A model for arts and health projects

In practice, if these principles are accepted, they lead to a different
way of thinking about, undertaking and evaluating arts projects
with social purposes, one based on a clear, common agreement of
values and objectives before work begins. It is a much more co-
operative, less hierarchical organisational model than those which
currently dominate in the mainstream of practice in medicine and
culture. It has five principal stages.

## Planning

Preliminary discussion and planning between all the project's
stakeholders (defined as anyone who can affect or be affected by its
work) are essential to clarify what problem, need or opportunity it
is designed to respond to. It may be that agreement is impossible at
this point – but how much better now than in a few months" time
after the investment of time, care, and resources? While there must
be a single common aim, for reasons already explained, it is
unrealistic to expect that all the objectives –  the subsidiary targets
to be achieved in meeting the aim – will be accorded equal
importance by all the stakeholders. A consultant will be primarily

concerned about the health aspects, while an artist will be more concerned about the quality of artwork produced; that should not be a problem where different aspirations are properly articulated and not incompatible.

## Identifying indicators and evaluation methods

When the aim and objectives of a project have been identified, it becomes relatively simple to identify the indicators which will show the extent to which original aspirations have been met. If a programme is expected to have an impact on people's health or quality of life, it will not be difficult to identify indicators in partnership with them which can show its outcomes; the Nottingham Health Profile mentioned above illustrates some of the possibilities.[5] More difficult is the question of how these indicators are to be measured – the evaluation methods. Questionnaires, whether self-administered or not, interviews, observation and more informal ideas like "comment walls", the use of tape or video recording all have a role to play (for examples, see Matarasso 1998).[11]

Some of these techniques, particularly questionnaires and structured interviews as well as health data such as levels of medication, will result in quantitative data, though the numbers involved in all but the largest studies must make us wary of its statistical reliability. There are also circumstances or outcomes which cannot be meaningfully quantified; for example, while one can ask participants about changes in their feelings and quantify the results, one can never be sure that the feelings they are reporting are equivalent and comparable. There will always be a balance to be struck between providing evidence which is required by the dominant ways of thinking and, precisely because this work is an extension to those existing paradigms, challenging the thinking itself.

The credibility of this type of data is evidently an issue in this context. My own view, based on extensive research, is that people are generally very reliable witnesses to change and think hard about their responses to it; there may be a tendency to be positive but it is not a significant factor. In any case, it seems to me to be difficult to discount people's own judgements of how they have benefited (or failed to benefit) from experiences they have had.

## Carrying out the work

Once the purpose of the project and the way it will be evaluated have been agreed, the work can go ahead, with data being recorded as it proceeds. Where change in people's health, feelings or quality of life is sought, it will be essential to create a profile of the situation before the start of the programme.

## Developing understanding of the results

At the end of the project, further data can be gathered and compiled. This is perhaps the most difficult part of the process for people who are engaged in evaluating their own projects, or for anyone not experienced in such work. This is most likely to be true of small-scale projects where the primary purpose is to develop understanding and practice within an institution or among a group of professionals rather than larger scale initiatives with the resources to bring in research time and skills. The most practical solution may be to see time spent discussing the interpretation of data as a valuable part not just of the evaluation but of the project itself. By exploring their different responses, the stakeholders can deepen their understanding of the project and its impact.

A word of warning, though, for projects which do have wider aspirations to affect policy or practice beyond their own environment. The public sector is overfond of the idea of models of good practice, widely reported as case studies, often failing to recognise the particular circumstances which made a project successful and what underlying factors would need to be mirrored before a project might be successfully replicated. As Nick Tilley has argued in the field of crime prevention: "Those undertaking demonstration projects, which are intended to yield transferable lessons, need so to write up their work that their conjectures concerning measures, mechanisms, context and outcome pattern are made explicit".[12]

## Reporting back and planning forward

The other element which is often neglected in existing approaches to evaluation is reporting back, especially to those who have contributed their thoughts, insights, and feelings as data for the evaluation. Without proper reporting back, people cannot learn from or respond to their experiences and initiatives therefore tend to be isolated occurrences rather than parts of a developing programme. Reporting back empowers those involved in a project by providing them with broader information and understanding than they can have as individuals and making it possible to move closer towards the principle of securing informed consent to change. Through it, a process becomes cyclical and enables the gradual transference of knowledge, understanding, and power between the stakeholders in a given activity.

## Processes, not solutions

It will be clear that evaluation should be seen as integral to any programme or initiative in the arts and health field, indeed in any similar type of activity, and that its needs and values have a direct bearing on the way such a project is thought about and carried out. The arts and humanities have a great deal to offer medicine and healthcare generally. Moreover, their contribution can be identified, expressed, and understood, enabling us to compare the value and cost-effectiveness of arts investment with other forms of intervention. If the processes by which we may do this are imperfect, they have that much in common with the practice of medicine or of art, and the imperfection matters less than that it should be recognised. We need to understand that there are no solutions to the complex challenges thrown up by questions of health, art, and human rights; the benefits lie in the way in which we manage the processes, not in some unattainable ideal. As Bernhard Schlink's philosopher concludes:

"No, your problem has no appealing solution. Of course one must act if the situation as you describe it is one of accrued or inherited responsibility. If one knows what is good for another person who in turn is blind to it, then one must try to open his eyes. One has to leave him the last word, but one must talk to him – to him and not to someone else behind his back."[1]

## References and notes

1 Schlink B. *The Reader* (trans. Janeway CB). London: Phoenix House, 1997.
2 Matarasso F. *Regular Marvels: a handbook for animateurs, practitioners and development workers in dance, mime, music and literature.* Leicester: Community Dance and Mime Foundation, 1994: 3–4.
3 Feynman RP. *The Meaning of It All.* London: Allen Lane, 1998:15
4 Seale C. The evaluation of health care. In: Davey B, Popay J (eds). *Dilemmas in Health Care.* Milton Keynes: Open University Press, 1993.
5 Hunt SM, McEwen J, McKenna SP. *Measuring Health Status.* London: Croom Helm, 1986.

6   Matarasso F. *Use or Ornament? The Social Impact of Participation in the Arts.* Stroud: Comedia, 1997.
7   Haldane D, Loppert S. *The Arts in health care: learning from experience.* London: King's Fund, 1999.
8   Hodges I, Norton V. *Artists at Stewart Villa.* Wellington, New Zealand: Department of Health, 1991.
9   Matarasso F. *Defining Values: evaluation in the arts.* Stroud: Comedia, 1996: 24.
10  Moriarty G. *Taliruni's Travellers: an arts worker's view of evaluation.* Stroud: Comedia, 1997: 17.
11  Matarasso F. *Poverty and Oysters: the social impact of local arts development in Portsmouth.* Stroud: Comedia, 1998.
12  Tilley N. *After Kirkholt: theory, method and results of replication evaluations.* London: Home Office, 1993: 19.

# 4

# Medical records as catalogues of experience

Anne Borsay

During the 1990s, a series of excellent histories of medicine were published in Britain, some the work of single authors and others edited or composite collections.[1] Lavishly illustrated popular studies also appeared, claiming to "enthral both layman and medical professional alike."[2] This chapter does not try to offer a miniature version of these encyclopaedic surveys. Rather, its purpose is to tease out the lessons of medical history for medical practice.

With this end in mind, four main themes are pursued. First, the intellectual stages through which history and medical history have passed are outlined. Second, the methodological consequences for the application of historical records are examined. Third, the changing doctor–patient relationship is used as a case study to illustrate how medical records have been used to catalogue experiences of medicine. And, finally, the implications of historical enquiry for healthcare practitioners are assessed in terms of both procedure and substance.

## History, social history and medicine

History as we know it today is a product of the modernisation process which by the 17th century was beginning to transform western Europe. Though the forces of transition were complex and varied, the intellectual rationalism of the Enlightenment played a central part. Tracing the source of all human misery to ignorance and superstition, Enlightenment thinking maintained that scientific knowledge would "pave the way for endless human progress."[3] Consequently, experience and experiment were privileged over the religious *a priori* reasoning which had underpinned the classical Renaissance and the Protestant Reformation, and secular sciences of man were shaped to inform strategies for personal and social improvement.[4] Enlightenment historiography thus turned to the past, seeking, in David Hume's words, "only to discover the constant and universal principles of human nature, by shewing men in all varieties of circumstances and situations."[5] Moreover, that endeavour was imbued with characteristic progressivism, well captured by Edward Gibbon in his *Decline and Fall of the Roman Empire* (1776–88); the English constitutional settlement of 1689, and the individual freedoms that resulted from the new relationship between monarch, Church, and Parliament, were celebrated "by chastising the Romans for having won the same prize and having lost it."[6]

The French Revolution of 1789 triggered a backlash against such abstract Enlightenment optimism and a retreat into empiricism which avoided political controversy. Principal among its architects was the German historian, Leopold von Ranke, whose long career spanned much of the 19th century. Ranke "merely want[ed] to show how, essentially, things happened"; for him, the "[s]trict presentation of facts, no matter how conditional and unattractive they might be, [wa]s undoubtedly the supreme law".[7] This disciplined methodology, to be achieved by a close and careful scrutiny of documentary records, was endorsed by early 19th century British historians who, like Thomas Macaulay, criticised their Enlightenment predecessors for giving "prominence to all the circumstances which support... [the] case... [and] glid[ing] lightly over those which are unfavourable to it". From the 1860s, however, there were attempts at a more systematic historiography. HT Buckle, an early proponent of the new approach, aimed to "accomplish for the history of man something equivalent, or at all events analogous, to what has been effected by the enquiries for the different branches of natural science". Consequently, the discipline needed urgent rescue from "the hands of biographers, genealogists and collectors of anecdotes, chroniclers of courts and princes and nobles". And in their place were required the categories and laws of human behaviour with which the Enlightenment had experimented.[8]

Buckle's own *History of the Civilization of England* (1857–61) met with an acrimonious reception. "The true historian takes the individual for his centre", thundered Lord Acton, Regius Professor of History at Cambridge, and "[i]f he treats of mobs, or armies, or bodies of men, he invests this multitude with a kind of personality of its own – its own wishes, passions, character, will, and conscience."[9] Despite this hostility, concepts and practices drawn initially from the natural and physical but later from the social sciences did make inroads into history and broaden its scope. Darwin's belief in the survival of the fittest, for example, spawned histories based on evolutionary ideas;[10] and the Marxist model fired by class conflict – as economic forces and social relations clashed to drive the transition from one mode of production to another – inspired a series of damning critiques of the Industrial Revolution and its social costs which continued into the 1930s.[11] A more explicit Marxist historiography was to blossom during the post-war period. Writers like Eric Hobsbawm, Christopher Hill and Edward Thompson were not crude economic determinists. On the contrary, they developed sophisticated arguments that were anchored in the detailed analysis of historical records.[12] Furthermore, Thompson's commitment, in *The Making of the English Working Class* (1963), "to rescue the poor...from the enormous condescension of posterity" was a seminal contribution to the emergence of social history as a mature subdiscipline.[13] The result was a more catholic agenda in which the everyday lives of ordinary people joined the dominant narrative of political elites.

The history of medicine broadly tracked the development of history as a whole, the grip of empiricism preserving a preoccupation with "great individuals" and "great events". In 1965 the British Society for the History of Medicine was established, with representatives from the history section of the Royal Society of Medicine, the Worshipful Society of Apothecaries, the Scottish Society for the History of Medicine and the Osler Club of London. The new society continued a long "tradition of gentlemanly scholarship exploring medicine's intellectual history and tracing the lives and careers of medicine's 'significant' men". However, it also promoted ventures into institutional and social history which reflected a more critical historiography, due in part to persistent difficulties with the National Health Service. This thrust was advanced by the foundation of the Society for the Social History of Medicine in 1970. The initial impetus for the SSHM came from teachers of public health history, anxious to expand the material for courses on offer to medical students, doctors following the public health diploma, and paramedical workers. Their attachment to the academic discipline of social medicine, set up in the 1940s "as a new pathway to identifying the health needs of the post-war world", was clearly reflected in the first mission statement.

> The aim of the Society is to promote a better understanding of the relationship between Medicine and the Social Sciences. Some knowledge of historical developments will further this aim and will bring together those engaged in academic and practical work such as doctors, sociologists, teachers and those engaged in public health, occupational medicine and community welfare services.

According to this agenda, history was "only marginally relevant to the Society's central purpose and direction", "a subordinate focus for shedding light on the medicine/social sciences interface."[14]

The "sociological approach" to the history of medicine was endorsed by Thomas McKeown, Professor of Social Medicine at Birmingham, when he gave the Society's inaugural lecture. The "social history of medicine was medical history with the 'public interest put in' "; it had to take an "operational approach"; most of all, it had to take its terms of reference "from the difficulties confronting medicine in the present day".[15] By 1976, however, this narrow definition of utility was under fierce scrutiny. In his Presidential Address of that year, Charles Webster argued forcefully for

> a deeper kind of relevance ... [which] emerges in the course of examining medicine from the perspective of the beliefs, values, social organization, and professional activities of every *stratum* within the ranks of medical practitioners; and by regarding patients as more than passive objects of disease. It should be an essential part of our brief to resurrect the patient, by contributing to the historical investigation of physical growth, mental development, and social customs – of all the conditions surrounding birth, and the events connected with death – of the state of health, and perceptions of disease of all classes within the population.

During the last 20 years, Webster's vision of a "medical history utilizing the values and techniques of the new 'social history' " has been realised.[16] Although the hagiographic or uncritically enthusiastic genre continues, professional historians of medicine are overwhelmingly dedicated to the broad contextualisation of their subject.

# From empiricism to social practice

If social history and the social history of medicine broke the political hegemony of the discipline, they perpetuated the neo-Rankean belief in an objective, empirical methodology. Acton, Ranke's most vocal devotee in Britain, insisted that the forensic scrutiny of documentary records enabled the historian "to repress the poet, the patriot, the religious or political partisan, to sustain no cause, to banish himself from his books". In 1931 Acton and his contemporaries were taken to task for failing to meet this benchmark; their promotion of a Whig version of constitutional history, argued Herbert Butterfield, was a progressive one which envisaged late Victorian Britain as the pinnacle of national and imperial achievement.[17] The triumphant flourish with which Mark Buer finished his 1926 volume on health, wealth and population between 1760 and 1815 demonstrates that medical history too had difficulty attaining Ranke's criteria: "We are yet on the threshold of the door which science and freeedom have opened", he enthused, "and the study of the last two centuries, viewed in the right perspective, leads, not to a paralysing pessimism, but to an optimism illumined by the brightest hopes for the future of mankind."[18]

Such breaches were attributed to professional shortcomings rather than to any inherent problems with objective history. In 1961, however, EH Carr launched an assault on empiricism, stressing that historical writings were coloured both by the personal characteristics of their authors – class, race, gender, age, politics – and by the contemporary societies which they inhabited. "When we attempt to answer the question 'What is history?'", he argued, "our answer, consciously or unconsciously, reflects our own position in time, and forms part of our answer to the broader question what view we take of the society in which we live".[19] Though the relationship between fact and value was "old hat" in the social sciences, Carr's call for a philosophy of history went unheeded. Indeed, his book provoked a robust reassertion of the conservative case. "But that men cannot ever eliminate themselves from the search for truth is nonsense", blasted GR Elton, "and pernicious nonsense at that, because it ... favours the purely relativist concept of history, the opinion that it is all simply in the historian's mind and becomes whatever he likes to make it".[20]

From the early 1990s, Elton's dogmatism incensed postmodernists who fixed their gaze on history. Rejecting the rationalism that was at the heart of the Enlightenment, their doctrine pronounces the death of modernity and the birth of a new era in which reason and reality are dethroned. The implications are too serious for historians to ignore. Postmodernism points up major changes in late 20th century society, notably the fragmentation arising from the relentless pursuit of consumerism and new information and communication technologies which even demote the individual self of modernist discourse into a mere subject.[21] Associated with this fracturing is a breakdown of all the metanarratives that underpinned modernity: Christianity, Marxism, progress and science.[22] The effect is to subvert historical time, rendering it meaningless. As Krishan Kumar explains:

> The post-modern rejection of grand narratives...devalues the past. The past is no longer a story within which we can situate ourselves – whether that story be one of growth, progress and emancipation, or one of growth, maturity and decline. We have no grounds for reading such significance in history....In the postmodernist view all periods are equal – equally full and equally empty, equally interesting and equally uninteresting.

What then fills the vacuum are "*simulacra*, images or representations of the past – but with no sense of the past that is represented".[23]

If history is created in the present rather than discovered in the past,[24] the pursuit of truth becomes futile. First, historical sources offer no direct access to historical reality; they are simply linguistic texts open to a multiplicity of fluid interpretations. Second, the discourses that emerge are politicised rather than objective. "We should admit...that power produces knowledge", wrote Michel Foucault, "that power and knowledge directly imply one another; that there is no power relation without the correlative constitution of a field of knowledge, nor any knowledge that does not presuppose and constitute at the same time power relations".[25] Postmodernism has done valuable service in flagging up the role of language and power in the construction of historical knowledge. To begin with, traditional sources are used with more imagination, documents being read for their linguistic and visual patterning as well as interrogated for their provenance – authenticity, reliability, authorship and purpose.[26] In addition, the emphasis on texts corrodes political, economic and social determinism, enables a constitutive role for cultural forms previously regarded as derivative or reflective,[27] and hence elevates the importance of those forms, so that historians now pay much greater attention to how the past is represented in art and architecture, literature and music, film, photography and heritage.[28]

Integral to these developments is a heightened awareness of the historian's positioning born of postmodernist sensitivities to knowledge as power. Paradoxically, this equation also poses fundamental dilemmas for historiography. Postmodernists market the ensuing "moral relativitism ... as the basis for social toleration and the positive recognition of differences".[29] But the risks are profound without a universal code which enshrines the human rights of minority groups.[30] Equally problematic is the accompanying "epistemological scepticism". Although British historians have tackled this issue,[5, 31] the most sustained response is to be found in an American study called *Telling the Truth About History* by Joyce Appleby, Lynn Hunt and Margaret Jacob.[15] The authors concede that objectivity, inspired by the heroic science of the 19th century with its neutral experimentation, is untenable. However, they resist the relativity of both language and knowledge. The solution to postmodernism's linguistic nihilism is through recourse to a new "practical realism".

> [T]he meanings of words are never simply "in our head", nor do they lock on to objects of the external world and fix reality for all time. Linguistic conventions arise because human beings possessed of imagination and understanding use language in response to things outside their minds. ... Communicative and responsive, words serve the goal of truth-seeking exactly because they are not the arbitrary tools of solipsists. Grammar may be deeply embedded in the human mind, but words result from contact with the world.

This potential for stable meanings opens the door to historical knowledge which is not utterly subjective. But since "all histories start with the curiosity of a particular individual and take shape under the guidance of his or her personal and cultural attributes",[32] how do we cope with the way in which political values inevitably intrude into any study of the past?

Postmodernism's reaction to the ubiquity of politics is a decentred model in which power is "local and unstable", "never in anybody's hands, never appropriated as a commodity or piece of wealth".[33] In practice, power is not free-floating but involves the structured domination of individuals, groups or classes; and under these circumstances, the liberal democracies characteristic of modernity offer better prospects for the toleration of difference.[34] In the case of history, a mechanical apparatus of footnotes for referencing sources not only allows each argument to be checked and evaluated but also articulates the moral imperative to conform to the approved rules of intellectual engagement.[35] Moreover, the pluralist ethos that underwrites liberal democracy nourishes an expectation of political freedom and choice which is consistent with historiographical divergence. Though this variety is incompatible with the search for one objective truth that underpinned empiricism, it accords with the notion of history as a contingent social practice. As Appleby and her colleagues conclude:

> The fact that there can be a multiplicity of accurate histories does not turn accuracy into a fugitive from a more confident age; it only points to the expanded necessity of men and women to read the many messages packed into a past event and to follow their different trajectories as that event's consequences concatenate through time.[36]

As for history, so for medical history. There may be no definitive answer lurking in the records, but competing interpretations of the medical past are a creative force when drawn up in accordance with the intellectual principles of liberal democracy.

## The medical marketplace

So far this chapter has identified medical history as a social practice, steering a middle way between the objectivity of empiricism and the subjectivity of postmodernism, to contextualise historical experiences of medicine. To appreciate the practical relevance of this activity, however, a concrete example of medical records under scrutiny is needed. Though the vibrancy of the field ensures no shortage of possibilities, we shall concentrate on the changing doctor–patient relationship during the 18th and early 19th centuries, a theme which demands consideration of the medical marketplace and the nature of medical knowledge and practice, as well as the patient interface itself. A spread of different sources will be deployed – census returns and newspapers, the diary and the letter, portraiture and statistics – to complement medical texts and clinical notes and to illustrate the richness of medical records at the historian's disposal.

Medicine in contemporary Britain is undertaken within an evolving European tradition which dates back to classical antiquity and its particular focus on the body. Drawing on the schematic work of Erwin Ackerknecht and Michel Foucault,[37] historical sociology in the 1970s posited a sequential model of transition from "bedside" to "hospital" medicine between the late 18th and early 19th centuries. Developed most comprehensively by ND Jewson, each "medical cosmology" was associated with its own forms of political economy, medical knowledge, and medical practice. In the bedside model, patients were fee-paying patrons, conceived of as sick persons with a "total psycho-somatic disturbance" which required heroic and extensive therapy based on qualitative diagnosis. In the hospital model, the institution or the state became the patron and patients were reduced to cases with "organic lesions", diagnosed through physical examination but treated minimally unless surgery was prescribed.[38]

Whilst this typology is a useful starting point for the doctor-patient relationship, recourse to the medical records suggests that it oversimplifies the political economy of medicine and the changing character of medical knowledge and practice. According to the bedside model, paying patients reigned supreme, bestowing their patronage in a medical marketplace where there was no theoretical or therapeutic consensus and hence a wide range of options to choose from. The diversity is indisputable. "Orthodox" practitioners were split into three categories. Physicians, governed by a Royal College dating back to 1518, dealt with internal disorders, tying their diagnoses to case histories which included observation of the patient as well as information about constitution and lifestyle. Surgeons, associated with the Barber-Surgeons' Company until they became a Royal College in 1800, carried out operations but more commonly treated wounds and fractures. Finally, apothecaries, members of the Grocers' Company before winning a Royal Charter in 1617, were responsible for compounding, supplying and selling drugs.[39]

Over and above these "orthodox" practitioners, census returns, newspaper advertisements, and medical directories show an array of "fringe" practitioners. In Bristol, for instance, 48 "irregular" (compared with 120 "regular") practitioners were picked up from these sources in the mid-19th century and this excluded nurses, midwives and those offering very specialist services (such as opticians and truss-makers) on the grounds that they were difficult to locate and classify. Practitioners who described their activities in some other way were also omitted.[40] Therefore, firms like the printers and publishers in the Lincolnshire town of Sleaford, who sold Fawcett's Pills with the help of a ditty promising a "perfect cure... [for] all your grief and ailing", escaped from view.[41]

These mid-Victorian purveyors of what we today call alternative medicine permitted the autonomous consumer of the bedside model to purchase these medical goods. At the other extreme, however, the micro-politics of the consultation were more subtle. Qualified practitioners, themselves increasingly wealthy, were not automatically intimidated even by their aristocratic clientele and although patients holding the purse strings were free to ignore advice, illness created a dependency that the doctor was able to exploit in his own financial interests. The net effect of these cross-currents was a "rough and ready parity" between clinician and patient, rather than the "quasi-monopolistic professional control" that was to thrive in the later Victorian period.[42]

## Medical knowledge

The political economy of 18th century medicine was linked with a distinctive epistemology in which "orthodox" practitioners enjoyed no monopoly over "fringe" remedies. The bedside model endowed this form of medical knowledge with "two major growth points": "phenomenological nosology" which defined disease "in terms of its external and subjective manifestations", and "speculative pathology" which neglected "proximate and precipitating causes" in favour of the "morbid forces" indicative of a "general underlying predisposition towards ill health". Consequently, the patient was envisaged as "a conscious human totality" in a way that transcended the divide between "psyche and soma found in modern medicine".[43] Printed medical texts betray an ongoing loyalty to the classical holism of Hippocrates and Galen consistent with this interpretation. Essentially, good health consisted of a stable balance of blood, phlegm, yellow bile, and black bile, the proper proportions of which varied according to age and personality.[44] Even before the Enlightenment, however, the humoral orthodoxy was losing credibility, the English physician William Harvey consolidating the challenge of Renaissance surgery with his theory of the circulation of the blood in 1616.[45]

The Scientific Revolution of the later 17th century led to further nuanced changes in medicine. Newton transformed the foundations of knowledge, his method of inducing general conclusions from experiment and observation combining with an innovative theoretical approach to construe matter as "particles... of different shapes, sizes and motions".[46] William Cullen (1710–90), Professor of Medicine at the University of Edinburgh, exemplifies the slow but sure adaptation. His *Synopsis Nosologiae Methodicae*, first published in 1769, was a classification of outward symptoms rather than an aspiring ontology.[47] Yet he believed that factors external to the individual constitution (such as climate, diet and effluvia) were the major cause of most diseases. And he also reconfigured humoralism with reference to material entities in his definition of "the MOVING EXTREMITIES of the nerves": "...so framed as to be capable of a peculiar contractility, and, in consequence of their situation and attachments, to be, by their contraction, capable of moving most of the solid and fluid parts of the body".[48] If its fundamentals were little altered, medical knowledge nonetheless reacted to scientific changes.

The concept of hospital medicine, said to have originated in post-Revolutionary Paris during the early decades of the 19th century, likewise requires appraisal against the historical record. In theory, medical knowledge addressed "the delineation of objective disease entities by means of correlating external symptoms with internal lesions." "Pathology took the form of local solidarism, focusing upon specific morbid events within the tissues rather than upon general disturbances of the constitutional system as a whole"; and symptoms thus became mere "secondary indicators of disease."[49] The mentality of hospital medicine is clearly visible in the two main works of the French surgeon, Marie François Xavier Bichat (1771–1802): *Traité des Membranes* (1799) and *Anatomie Générale* (1801). "The more one will observe diseases and open cadavers," he wrote, "the more one will be convinced of the necessity of considering local diseases not from the aspect of the complex organs but from that of the individual tissues." Certainly, the influence of tissue pathology spread. In Britain, however, though developments in surgery represented a significant departure from humoralism, they were based on the individual organs and hence derived from earlier ideas of Padua's Professor of Anatomy, Giovanni Battista Morgagni (1682–1771).[50]

# Medical practice

Telling the story of medical knowledge from key texts throws into sharp relief the peaks of theoretical achievement but underplays how these ideas were received and implemented. Before the ascent of bacteriology, medical knowledge had few implications for health because medical practice was largely ineffective. However, methods of diagnosis and therapy did alter and so it is important to chart these changes and ask whether they affected medicine's therapeutic competence and effectiveness.

A perusal of the medical records brings to light a more complex picture than the shift from qualitative diagnosis and heroic, extensive treatments under the bedside model to physical examination and therapeutic scepticism under the hospital model.[51] Painted in 1891, Luke Fildes portrait of *The Doctor* personifies bedside medicine. The work depicts a doctor watching over a sick child, who lies across two mismatched chairs in a humble abode with anxious parents in the background. It was much acclaimed by the medical profession. "What do we not owe to Mr Fildes", declared one practitioner in the *British Medical Journal*, "for showing to the world the typical doctor, as we would all like to be shown – an honest man and a gentleman, doing his best to relieve suffering? A library of books written in our honour would not do what this picture has done and will do for the medical profession in making the hearts of our fellow-men warm to us with confidence and affection."[52] Yet though the portrait was in the same realist tradition that informed later 19th century British historiography, it was no more factual or objective.

The very act of representing three-dimensional space on a two-dimensional plane involves interpretation mediated through paint and technique.[53] That cultural process occurred against a commercial backdrop, the painting being commissioned by Sir Henry Tate for £3000 just before he donated his art collection to the nation. Fildes himself chose the subject, inspired by the death of his eldest son. However, he constructed a mock-up cottage interior in his studio, employed a professional model as the doctor and put together a composite image of the child from his own surviving children.[54] Furthermore, both the sponsorship of the patron and the decisions of the artist were socioculturally situated. Indebted to empiricism, Victorian realism embraced the modern world by responding democratically to the problems of industrialisation. Doctors, "nineteenth-century heroes in the service of humanity", were thus depicted "in their working milieu, in the midst of ... missions of mercy [to the poor]".[55] Luke Fildes' portrait must be read in this light as the product of a multi-faceted social practice. Such an interpretation does not deny that the ideal physicianly encounter occurred. What it suggests is that artistic representations of medicine cannot be reduced to unproblematic, transparent images of professional reality.

Experiences of the medical encounter recorded in diaries and letters are no less constructed, their authors engaged in interpretative processes independent of any intention to mislead. However, such sources do allow a comparison of perspectives within the doctor–patient relationship. In 1810, the novelist, Fanny Burney, underwent a mastectomy, performed without anaesthetic. Her harrowing account of the operation is widely quoted.

M. Dubois placed me upon the mattress, & spread a cambric handkerchief upon my face. It was transparent, however, & I saw through it that the bed stead was instantly surrounded by the 7 men and my nurse, I refused to be held; but when, bright through the cambric, I saw the glitter of polished steel – I closed my eyes ...

Yet – when the dreadful steel was plungd into the breast – cutting through veins – arteries – flesh – nerves – I needed no injunctions not to restrain my cries. I began a scream that lasted unintermittingly during the whole time of the incision – & I almost marvel that it rings not in my ears still! so excruciating was the agony. When the wound was made, & the instrument was withdrawn, the pain seemed undiminished, for the air that suddenly rushed into those delicate parts felt like a mass of minute but sharp & forked poniards, that were tearing the edges of the wound, but when again I felt the instrument –describing a curb – cutting against the grain, if I may so say, while the flesh resisted in a manner so forcible as to oppose & tire the hand of the operator, who was forced to change from the right to the left – then, indeed, I thought I must have expired, I attempted no more to open my eyes ... The instrument this second time withdrawn, I concluded the operation over – Oh no! presently the terrible cutting was renewed – & worse than ever, to separate the bottom, the foundation of this dreadful gland from the parts to which it adhered ... yet again all was not over.[56]

Contrast this with a diary entry by Richard Kay, a general

practitioner from Baldingstone near Bury in Lancashire. On 7 June 1749, Dr Kay visited Mrs Driver whose cancerous breast he had removed in December of the previous year.

[T]he wound cured, and she has been hearty some months; last Saturday she came here ... to show us a knot she had discovered that morning about an inch and a half below the old wound upon the forepart of her ribs, which growing so fast upon the Sunday, Monday, &c. Mrs Driver came here for us she being determined to undergo a second amputation, upon dissecting the knot I soon found I had more work to do than was expected as there appeared other kernels closely joined together which lay down to the abdomen and the compass of six or seven inches square, in some parts I took off the skin, in others dissected them from under the skin, so that below where her breast formerly was down her ribs to her belly I dissected from her at a moderate computation five hundred different distinct... knots or young cancers; she was sick and very poorly after the operation. I lodge at Mr Driver's. Lord, may we have hope towards God and may this support and comfort us under the different occurrences in life, yea under the severest afflictions and death itself.

Further surgery failed to save Mrs Driver and she was buried on 20 February 1750. Richard Kay attended the funeral, no doubt a mark of his professional dedication which was underscored by a strong Nonconformist faith and witnessed by long hours and much travel on horseback to care for patients. Yet Richard Kay's diary conveys no sense that the operation was conducted without effective pain relief.[57]

Although these instances of heroic surgery dramatise the psychological distance between doctor and patient, they convey a misleading impression of the medical practices to which most patients were exposed. General practitioners working in the community largely confined themselves to "minor surgery, local applications, and medicine". Take William Pulsford, a young surgeon in partnership with his uncle in the Somerset town of Wells. Of his 334 new cases listed in a ledger for 1757, only two involved a major operation, compared with 91 accidents, 35 sore throats, 31 sore legs, and 25 boils and abscesses.[58]

Prior to the administration of anaesthetics from the 1840s, hospital practice was not dissimilar. The voluntary infirmaries opening in Britain from the third decade of the 18th century pursued a complex series of economic, sociocultural and political goals in organising charitable assistance for the sick poor.[59] However, their publicity material, some of which survives in periodicals and newspapers, also advertised an educational role for the medical profession. The voluntary hospital "was of infinite use to all other persons as well as the poor", insisted a statement in the *Gentleman's Magazine* for 1741, "by furnishing the physicians and surgeons with more experience in one year, than they could have in ten without it".[60] The same argument was rehearsed in the proposal for an Exeter hospital which appeared in the *Bath Journal* 10 years later.[61]

Yet despite this pedagogic commitment, treatment regimes were conservative and the printed rules which governed the conduct of hospitals construed major surgery as an exceptional event. At the Leeds Infirmary, for example, "no amputation or other great operation, except an urgent occasion require it, [was to] be performed, without a previous consultation of the physicians and surgeons".[62] A manuscript case book for the early 1780s, containing 122 histories for in- and outpatients mainly treated by the Infirmary's senior surgeon, William Hey, suggests that this regulation was rarely invoked. There were three diagnoses of cancer, two compound fractures of the leg, one bladder stone, one fractured skull and one strangulated hernia. However, these figures were overrun by 34 cases of ague and 15 of rheumatism.[63]

Such chronic disease profiles, allied to the infrequent practice of major surgery, would seem to refute extravagant claims that voluntary hospitals were "gateways to death" during the 18th century.[64] The routine statistics published by the institutions in their *annual reports* endorse this conclusion. Thus at the Shrewsbury and Liverpool Infirmaries, patient mortality only rarely exceeded 7% per annum over the long 18th century.[65] Indeed, a survey of 117 hospitals in England and Wales, carried out in 1863 after the arrival of anaesthesia but immediately before Lister's revolutionary principles were introduced to deal with sepsis, yielded a surgical death rate of 12.51% after operations to the eye were excluded.[66] Of course, charities heavily dependent upon voluntary gifts had a vested interest in presenting their clinical activities in the most positive light. At the same time, however, the moral economy which they inhabited imposed expectations of propriety that were breached with peril. Consequently, it is safe to assume that printed statistics are a broadly reliable indicator of low hospital mortality.[67]

# The doctor–patient relationship

But if continuity rather than change was a feature of both bedside and hospital practice until the surgical revolution of the late 19th century, this does not necessarily imply that the doctor–patient relationship was static. Taking Bristol as her example, Mary Fissell has argued that the patient narrative was disappearing from hospital consultations after 1750. Her main sources are two sets of case histories: the manuscript notes of a surgeon called Alexander Morgan who worked in the city during the 1740s, and an 1816 *Compendium of Cases from the Bristol Infirmary* based on the work of James Bedingfield who was first the apothecary but later a surgeon. See how Morgan describes a patient with giddiness and head pains.

> The third day after the weather happened to be very warm he changed his thick waistcoat for a linen one & being careless sat a quarter day in a room that was wet the same evening he found himself not well & a little feverish & thirsty for which he went to bed and drank plentiful of sack whey. The next morning he was very hoarse and out of order...

Compare this with Bedingfield's account of a boy in hospital:

> His appearance was florid, his complexion clear. He complained of a slight headache and a sore throat. His pulse was full and rather frequent, the tongue white, the tonsils slightly inflamed, the parotid glands were very much enlarged, the bowels were confined, and there was a little oppression about the chest.

It is important not to overstate the differences between these two case histories. After all, Bedingfield did think fit to record his patient's stated ailments. But unlike Morgan, he abandoned the humoral practice of locating the particular illness within its environmental context. Instead, reliance was placed on "signs and symptoms" that were conducive to "disease-orientated diagnosis".[68] In the hospital, therefore, "objective" physical examination was dislodging "subjectively defined sensations and feelings", even before the invention of the stethoscope in 1816. Moreover, in an institution where patients faced ignominious dismissal for misbehaviour or dissent, treatment became non-negotiable and standardised into "an anti-phlogistic regimen [of] bleeding, purging, blisters, and a bland diet".[69] The upshot was a widening gulf between patient perceptions and medical knowledge and practice well in advance of Parisian hospital medicine.

The demise of the holistic patient narrative was consolidated in the late 19th century as cells and bacteria disclosed their secrets to the microscope and supplied a scientific platform for the launch of modern biomedicine. Show no sympathy to the poor, one London house physician told his medical students in 1899, for to do so was to invite "long-winded and totally unimportant details concerning the manner they received their injuries".[70] This advice came less than a decade after Luke Fildes" portrait of the caring doctor. It would be facile to explain the disparity solely in terms of the hospital/community axis for historical experiences catalogued from medical records demonstrate that the patient relationship was hotly contested territory.

## Learning from the past

Modern healthcare practitioners today continue their long tradition of writing medical history, the study of the past functioning as a humanistic recreation which complements their scientifically informed professional work. The relevance of historical analysis to contemporary practice is more controversial. Neither empiricists nor postmodernists are enthusiastic about learning from the past in any sphere, the former fearing a contamination of the objective truth[71] and the latter believing that without truth there can be no guide to future action.[72] Moreover, when the General Medical Council reviewed undergraduate education for *Tomorrow's Doctors* in the early 1990s, the value of history was recognised only in relation to "advances" in "medical research"; as Mark Jackson has observed, "[t]he humanities... are to remain faithful foot-soldiers in the war against disease, a war to be fought exclusively in the name of medical science."[73] Conceptualised as a social practice, however, medical history offers medical practice a menu of uses which extends beyond clinical research to medical epistemology and professional reflexivity.

There are occasions on which medical records are of direct relevance to clinical practice or research. Oral history, for instance, can be used to build the self-esteem of former inmates of mental deficiency institutions.[74] "I'd just like people to know", explained one ex-patient, "so they can realize what it was we'd had to go through. It's not true what was written down! They did it just to keep us locked up, so that people would think we're mental!"[75] Such qualitative experiences are salient to the quantitative search for medical knowledge which harnesses historical data to study the trajectories of genetically transmitted diseases or the impact of new drug regimes. In the West Midlands, for example, the links between sudden deaths in psychiatric hospitals and the prescription of antipsychotic medication are being investigated using patient notes from 1987 to 1997.[76]

There are also spin-offs for medical administration. Thus, a newly funded investigation of the Aberdeen typhoid outbreak in 1964 hopes to examine "the process by which the official report was produced . . . and look at why some things were implemented and others weren't". Professor Hugh Pennington, who chaired the recent Lanarkshire *E.coli* enquiry, is confident that the Aberdeen project, with which he is also associated, "will have direct relevance to the current situation."[77] Accepting that the past has a bearing on the present is not to subscribe to a crude, predictive model of history.[78] But though drawing analogies may deepen the comprehension of contemporary problems, "nothing in human society . . . ever happens twice under exactly the same conditions or in exactly the same way". Consequently, the past is better consulted to enhance the "depth and range of our understanding of the present" than trawled for "the solution to current problems".[79]

Conceived of in this more ambitious way, medical history is liberated from a prison of relevance which confines it to 20th century issues with contemporary epistemological or administrative connections. While postmodernism exaggerates the fragmentation of modern life, globalisation and technology, geographical mobility and occupational instability have weakened the conventional, ascribed roots of identity and placed a greater burden upon individuals to build and acquire their own personae;[80] it is no longer enough to be a doctor or a nurse or a health visitor, each person has to thrash out what the role means for them. The professional reflexivity, or critical thinking, that this requires is a lesson which history can help to teach by encouraging practitioners to draw methodological parallels between the construction of medical and historical knowledge, and to engage with the continuities and changes which characterise medical practices in their socio-historical contexts. Biomedicine and empirical history in Britain come from the same intellectual stable. However, both are social practices which benefit from acknowledging their democratic setting and the dangers of authoritarian alternatives; after all, neither discipline fared well in Nazi Germany or Stalinist Russia.

Like historians making sense of medical records, clinicians conscious of the philosophical spaces between evidence-based medicine and the individual patient have to weigh up the arguments but reconcile themselves to the uncertainty of no single input or outcome. And in becoming aware of the multifarious sources that feed into historical decision making – not just scientific but economic, social, political, and cultural – medicine is alerted to the multidisciplinary qualities of its own practice. "Blessed are they that considereth the poor and needy," sang out Handel's *Anthem for the Founding Hospital*. If this music constructed affluent 18th century benefactors as worthy and charitable, then 20th century attitudes to insanity are likewise constituted by Peter Maxwell Davies" *Eight Songs for a Mad King* or Alan Bennett's screenplay for *The Madness of King George*.

Thinking about the methodological ramifications of historical enquiry fuses into the substantive lessons for professional reflexivity. Our case study of the doctor–patient relationship immediately generates food for thought. Does a medical marketplace convey genuine choice and protect consumer interests? Is biomedicine able to treat the patient holistically, and would it be advantageous to do so? Why is job satisfaction a problem for the National Health Service when the morale of 18th century doctors apparently survived despite the lack of effective remedies? What does consent to agonising surgery tell us about patients' attitudes to pain? Are empathy and professionalism incompatible? What makes the hospital an intimidating environment? How do popular perceptions of medicine arise? And are there risks in taking for granted the advantages which scientific medicine bestows? None of these questions has easy answers. However, tackling them with a historical understanding casts old issues in a new light. First, it gives perspective by demonstrating that the present is but a temporary phase in an evolving chronology. Second, it testifies to the contextualisation of medicine. Neither medical knowledge nor medical practice operates in a vacuum. Both are socially contingent.[81] Therefore, it is no coincidence that the multiplicity of theories and therapies accommodated by 18th century humoralism was associated with a commercial medical marketplace and that the most sustained incursions against patient autonomy were made in charitable institutions where the sick poor had little power to resist.

# Conclusion

In this chapter, history has been characterised as a social practice rather than an objective quest for truth. The implication is that medical records do not simply catalogue or chronicle the past but lend themselves to competing interpretations, all of which may be accurate if disciplined by the rational conventions consistent with the freedoms and choices of liberal democracy. The application of this approach has been illustrated through a case study of the doctor–patient relationship. By no means every type of medical record has been included; Acts of Parliament, parliamentary debates and local government papers,[82] the national series of demographic statistics,[83] the visual imagery of documentary film and photography,[84] the architecture and geography of medical institutions,[85] the artefacts of prehistoric surgery,[86] and even the iconography of modern heritage sites[87] are all casualties of omission. Nonetheless, the changing interface between doctors and patients explored through a historical telescope reveals procedural dilemmas similar to the uncertainties of clinical decision making and substantive issues that resonate with contemporary problems. The professional reflexivity that results from this awareness is the principal aid that medical history offers to medical practice. To ensure that it remains a resource for future generations, long-term policies to preserve medical records, and short-term strategies to save material on the verge of destruction, are essential.[88]

# References and notes

1   See, for example, Porter R. *The Greatest Benefit to Mankind: a Medical History of Humanity from Antiquity to the Present*. London: HarperCollins, 1997; Conrad LI, Neve M, Nutton V, Porter R, Wear A. *The Western Medical Tradition 800 BC to AD 1800*. Cambridge: Cambridge University Press, 1995; Loudon I (ed.). *Western Medicine: An Illustrated History*, Oxford: Oxford University Press, 1997; Porter R (ed.). *The Cambridge Illustrated History of Medicine*. Cambridge: Cambridge University Press, 1996.

2   See, for example, Margotta R. *The Hamlyn History of Medicine*. London: Reed International, 1996, dust jacket.

3   Hollinger R. *Postmodernism and the Social Sciences: A Thematic Approach*. California: Sage, 1994: p. 7.

4   Dunthorne H. *The Enlightenment*. London: Historical Association, 1991: pp. 5–13; Porter R. *The Enlightenment*. Basingstoke: Macmillan, 1990, pp. 1–11, 18–20, 68–9.

5   Warren J. *The Past and Its Presenters: An Introduction to Issues in Historiography*. London: Hodder and Stoughton, 1998, p. 92.

6   Bentley M. *Modern Historiography: An Introduction*. London: Routledge, 1999, pp. 13–15.

7   Warren, *Past and its Presenters*, pp. 106–7.

8   Bentley, *Modern Historiography*, pp. 26, 48.

9   Bentley, *Modern Historiography*, p. 48.

10  See, for example, Traill HD and Mann JS, *Social England*, 7 vols London: Cassell, 1895.

11  See, for example, A Toynbee, *Lectures on the Industrial Revolution of the Eighteenth Century in England*, 1st Pub. 1884. London: Longmans, Green and Co., 1913; Hammond JL and B, *The Bleak Age*, 1st pub. 1934. West Drayon: Penguin, 1947.

12  Warren, *Past and Its Presenters*, pp. 138–46.

13  Thompson EP, *The Making of the English Working Class*. Harmondsworth: Penguin, 1963, p. 13.

14  Porter D, The Mission of Social History of Medicine: An Historical Overview, *Social History of Medicine*, 1995; **8**, 345–8.

15  McKeown T, 'A Sociological Approach to the History of Medicine', *Medical History*, 1970; **14**: 342.

16  Porter, Mission of Social History of Medicine, p. 351.

17  Warren, *Past and Its Presenters*, pp. 114, 117-20.

18  Buer MC, *Health, Wealth and Population in the Early Days of the Industrial Revolution*, London: George Routledge, 1926, p. 243.

19  Carr EH, *What Is History?* Harmondsworth: Penguin, 1961, p. 8.

20  Elton GR, *The Practice of History*, London: Collins, 1969, p. 77.

21  Appleby J, Hunt L and Jacob M, *Telling the Truth About History*, New York: W.W. Norton, 1994, p. 202; Lyon D, *Postmodernity*. Buckingham: Open University Press, 1994, p. 7; Sarup M, *An Introductory Guide to Post-Structuralism and Postmodernism*, 2nd edn Hemel Hempstead: Harvester Wheatsheaf, 1993, p. 181.

22  Jenkins K, *Re-Thinking History*, London: Routledge, 1991, pp. 60, 63; Munslow A, *Deconstructing History*, London: Routledge, 1997, pp. 14–15.

23  Kumar K, *From Post-Industrial to Post-Modern Society: New Theories of the Contemporary World*, Oxford: Blackwell, 1995, p. 145. See also Appleby *et al*, *Telling the Truth*, p. 205.

24  Jenkins, *Re-Thinking History*, pp. 32–3; Munslow, *Deconstructing History*, p. 178.

25  Foucault M, *Discipline and Punish: The Birth of the Prison*, trans. by Sheridan A, 1st pub. 1975. Harmondsworth: Penguin, 1977, p. 27.

26  Marwick A, *The Nature of History*, London: Macmillan, 1970. pp. 136-7.

27  Evans RJ, *In Defence of History*, London: Granta, 1997, pp. 243–4; Kumar, *From Post-Industrial to Post-Modern Society*, pp. 101–2; Leonard P, *Postmodern Welfare: Reconstructing an Emancipatory Project*, London: Sage, 1997, pp. 1–2.

28  Evans, *In Defence of History*, p. 244.

29  Jenkins, *Re-Thinking History*, pp. 56, 66. See also Southgate B, *History: What and Why? Ancient, Modern and Postmodern Perspectives*, London: Routledge, 1996, p. 133

30  Eagleton T, *The Illusions of Postmodernism*, Oxford: Blackwell, 1996, pp. 123, 134–5; Evans, *In Defence of History*, pp. 184-5.

31  The most robust rebuttal is Evans, *In Defence of History*. See also Warren, *The Past and Its Presenters*, pp. 13–23.

32  Appleby *et al*, *Telling the Truth About History*, pp. 247–8, 254, 260.

33  Gordon C (ed.), *Michel Foucault Power/Knowledge: Selected Interviews and Other Writings 1972–1977*, Brighton: Harvester, 1980, p. 98; Foucault M, *The History of Sexuality*, trans. by Hurley R, 3 vols Harmondsworth: Penguin, 1981, I: *An Introduction*, p. 94.

34  Eagleton, *Illusions of Postmodernism*, pp. 76–80, 85–92.

35  For a philosophical defence of rationality as a universal good, see S. Hampshire, *Innocence and Experience*, London: Allen Lane, 1989.

36  Appleby *et al*, *Telling the Truth About History*, pp. 261–2.

37  Ackerknecht EH, *Medicine at the Paris Hospital 1794–1848*, Baltimore: John Hopkins Press, 1967; Foucault M, *The Birth of the Clinic: An Archaeology of*

*Medical Perception*, 1st pub. 1963, trans by A.M. Sheridan, repr. London: Routledge, 1989.

38  Jewson ND. The Disappearance of the Sick Man from Medical Cosmology, 1770–1870, *Medical History*, 1976; 10: 227–30.

39  Loudon I, *Medical Care and the General Practitioner 1750–1850*, Oxford: Clarendon Press, 1986, p. 19; Peterson MJ, *The Medical Profession in Mid-Victorian London*, Berkeley: University of California Press, 1978, pp. 6, 9, 11.

40  Brown PS, The Providers of Medical Treatment in Nineteenth-Century Bristol, *Medical History*, 1980; **24**: 313.

41  Ellis C, The Old, the Sick and the Poor, in Ellis C (ed.), *Mid Victorian Sleaford 1851–1871*, Lincoln: Lincolnshire Library Service, 1981, p. 167.

42  Porter D and Porter R, *Patient's Progress: Doctors and Doctoring in Eighteenth-Century England*, Cambridge: Polity, 1989, pp. 95, 208.

43  Jewson, Disappearance, pp. 227–9.

44  Jewson ND, Medical Knowledge and the Patronage System in Eighteenth-Century England, *Sociology*, 1974; **8**: 371–2.

45  Porter, *Greatest Benefit*, pp. 211–16.

46  Wear A, Making Sense of Health and the Environment in Early Modern England, in Wear A (ed.), *Medicine in Society: Historical Essays* Cambridge: Cambridge University Press, 1992, p. 120.

47  Porter, *Greatest Benefit*, pp. 260–2; Risse G, *Hospital Life in Enlightenment Scotland: Care and Teaching at the Royal Infirmary of Edinburgh*, Cambridge: Cambridge University Press. 1986, pp. 116–17.

48  Bynum WF, Cullen and the Nervous System, in Doig A, Ferguson JPS, Milne IA and Passmore R (eds), *William Cullen and the Eighteenth-Century Medical World*, Edinburgh: University of Edinburgh Press, 1993, p. 157. See also Risse GB, Medicine in the Age of Enlightenment, Wear A (ed.), *Medicine in Society: Historical Essays*, Cambridge: Cambridge University Press, 1992, pp. 163–4.

49  Jewson, Disappearance, pp. 229–30.

50  Porter, *Greatest Benefit*, pp. 263–5, 307.

51  Jewson, 'Disappearance', p. 228.

52  *British Medical Journal*, 8 October 1892, pp. 787–8.

53  Nochlin L, *Realism*, Harmondsworth: Penguin, 1971, pp. 14–15.

54  Treuherz J, *Hard Times: Social Realism in Victorian Art*, London: Lund Humphries and New York: Moyer Bell, in association with Manchester City Art Galleries, 1987, pp. 86–9.

55  Nochlin L, *Realism*, pp. 17, 23–5, 28, 33, 192.

56  Porter, *Greatest Benefit*, p. 365.

57  Brockbank W and Kenworthy F (eds), *The Diary of Richard Kay, 1716–51 of Baldingstone, near Bury: A Lancashire Doctor*, Manchester: Chetham Society, 1968, pp. 134, 135, 136, 141–2, 146, 147, 151.

58  Loudon, *Medical Care*, pp. 74, 76, 78–9.

59  See, for example, Borsay A, *Medicine and Charity in Georgian Bath: A Social History of the General Infirmary c1739–1830*, Aldershot: Ashgate, 1999; Borsay A, Cash and Conscience: Financing the General Hospital at Bath, c.1739–1750, *Social History of Medicine*, 1991; 4: 207–29: Borsay A, 'Returning Patients to the Community: Disability, Medicine and Economic Rationality Before the Industrial Revolution', *Disability and Society*, 1998; **13**: 645-63; Borsay A, 'A Middle Class in the Making: The Negotiation of Power and Status at Bath's Early Georgian General Infirmary, c.1739–1765, *Social History*, 1999; **24**: 269–86. Almost 40 institutions had been founded in England and Scotland by 1800. See J Woodward, *To Do the Sick No Harm: A Study of the Voluntary Hospital System to 1875*, London: Routledge and Kegan Paul, 1974, pp. 147–8.

60  A View of the Many Peculiar Advantages of Public Hospitals, *Gentleman's Magazine*, 1741; **XI** 476–7.

61  *Bath Journal*, 14 January 1751.

62  Anning ST, *The General Infirmary at Leeds*, 2 vols Edinburgh and London: E. & S. Livingstone, 1963–6, I: *The First Hundred Years 1767–1869*, 1963, p. 33.

63  Anning ST, A Medical Case Book: Leeds. 1781–84, *Medical History*, 1984; **28**: 420–1.

64  Helleiner KF, 'The Vital Revolution Reconsidered', *Canadian Journal of Economics and Political Science*, 1957; XXIII: 6.

65  A Comparative Average Statement of In and Out-Patients, in Bevan H, *Records of the Salop Infirmary from the Commencement of the Charity to the Present Time*, Shrewsbury, 1847; McLoughlin G, *A Short History of the First Liverpool Infirmary 1749–1824*, London and Chichester: Phillimore, 1978, pp. 101–3, Appendix IX.

66  Woodward, *To Do the Sick No Harm*, pp. 81–2.

67  Borsay A, "Persons of Honour and Reputalion": The Voluntary Hospital in an Age of Corruption, *Medical History*, 1991;**35**: 281–94; Borsay A, An Example of Political Arithmetic: The Evaluation of Spa Therapy at the Georgian Bath Infirmary. 1742–1830, *Medical History* 2000; **44**: 149–72.

68  Fissel ME, The Disappearance of the Patient's Narrative and the Invention of Hospital Medicine, in French R and Wear A (eds), *British Medicine in an Age of Reform*, London: Routledge, 1991, pp. 92–106.

69  Jewson, Disappearance, pp. 229–30.

70  *British Medical Journal*, 23 September 1899, p. 797.

71  Tosh J, *The Pursuit of History: Aims, Methods and New Directions in the Study of Modern History*, 2nd edn London: Longman, 1991, p. 25.

72  Warren, *The Past and Its Presenters*, p. 5.

73  Jackson M, Medical Humanities in Medical Education, *Medical Education*, 1996; **30**: 396.

74  Stevens A, Recording the History of an Institution: The Royal Eastern Counties Institution at Colchester, in Atkinson D, Jackson M and Walmsley J, *Forgotten Lives: Exploring the History of Learning Disability*, Kidderminster: British Institute of Learning Disabilities, 1997, p. 48.

75  Fido R and Pott M, Using Oral Histories, in Atkinson D, Jackson M and Walmsley J, *Forgotten Lives: Exploring the History of Learning Disability*, Kidderminster: British Institute of Learning Disabilities, 1997, p. 45.

76  Hidden Evidence: Sudden Death and Antipsychotics, *Wellcome News*, 1999; **18**: 20.

77  Aberdeen Anguish: The Aberdeen Typhoid Outbreak of 1964, *Wellcome News*, 1999; **18**: 16–17.

78  Evans, *In Defence of History*, p. 59.

79  Tosh. *Pursuit of History*, pp. 9–20.

80  Giddens A, *Modernity and Self-Identity: Self and Society in the Late Modern Age*, Cambridge: Polity, 1991, 1–9.

81  Jackson, Medical Humanities, pp. 395–6; Jackson M, The Use of Historical Study in Medical Research, *Family Practice*, 1996; **13**: Supplement 1, S17–20.

82  See, for example, Thomson M, *The Problem of Mental Deficiency: Eugenics. Democracy and Social Policy in Britain c.1870–1959*, Oxford: Clarendon Press, 1998.

83  See, for example, Szreter S, The Importance of Social Intervention in Britain's Mortality Decline c.1850–1914: A Re-interpretation of the Role of Public Health, *Social History of Medicine*, 1; 1988: 1–37.

84  See, for example, Jackson M. 'Images of Deviance: Visual Representations of Mental Defectives in Early Twentieth-Century Medical Texts', *British Journal for the History of Science*, **28**; 1995: 319–37.

85  See, for example, Markus T, *Buildings and Power: Freedom and Control in the Origin of Modern Building Types*, London: Routledge, 1993; Philo C, "Enough to Drive One Mad": The Organization of Space in Nineteenth-Century Lunatic Asylums, in Wolch J and Dear M (eds), *The Power of Geography: How Territory*

*Shapes Social Life*, Boston: Unwin Hyman, 1989, pp. 258–90.

86  See, for example, Arnott R, 'Healing and Medicine in the Aegean Bronze Age', *Journal of the Royal Society of Medicine*, **89**; 1996: 265–9.

87  See, for example, Arnold K, 'Birth and Breeding: Politics on Display at the Wellcome Institute for the History of Medicine', in Macdonald S (ed.), *The Politics of Display: Museums, Science, Culture*, London: Routledge, 1998, pp. 183–96.

88  Higgs E and Melling J, Chasing the Ambulance: The Emerging Crisis in the Preservation of Modern Health Records, *Social History of Medicine*, **10**; 1997: 127–36; Sabovic Z and Pearson D (eds), *A Healthy Heritage: Collecting for the Future of Medical History – Conference Proceedings*, London: Wellcome Trust, 1999.

# Section 2
# Patients and professionals

| | | |
|---|---|---:|
| *Introduction* | | 77 |
| 5 | The consultation as Rubik's cube | 83 |
| 6 | The new genetics: retelling and reinterpreting an old story | 101 |
| 7 | Poetry as a key for healthcare | 119 |
| 8 | Spirituality as an integral part of healthcare | 136 |

# Introduction

Medicine, and healthcare more generally, are primarily constituted by the interactions between individual human beings, be they patients or practitioners. These interactions are usually of a special kind, heavily influenced both by the consequences of illness, diagnosis, and management and by the institutional and technological backdrop against which the interaction is played out – be it an anxious initial consultation, a postoperative assessment, a counselling session, a rehabilitation exercise or, sometimes, the making comfortable of a dying patient. Accordingly this section focuses on professional and lay perspectives on the clinical interaction and particularly upon the place of experience and how experiences are interpreted – whether by practitioners or by patients. It could be said that the humanities disciplines, taken together, are themselves centrally concerned with the recording and interpretation of experiences. If this is true, then the *medical* humanities are centrally concerned with the recording and interpretation of experiences of medical and healthcare.

Kieran Sweeney is a general practitioner in a family practice established in the mould of the long-term, continual care of succeeding generations of local people. He considers and challenges some aspects of the orthodox model of evidence-based primary medical care and suggests an alternative model in which fuller account is taken of the diversity of patients' – and practitioners" – experiences and interpretations of health, illness, and the clinical encounter. The different forms of language, vocabulary and explanatory frameworks, which are variously at the disposal of patients and professionals, underlie the questions explored by another general practitioner, Deborah Kirklin, in connection with one of the most significant areas of medical science, the "genetic revolution". Kirklin is concerned with the influences at work in how patients and professionals conceptualise, evaluate and above all *experience* the implications of the new technology.

The interpretation of experience is of course at the root of artistic and literary expression. Gillie Bolton is a professional creative writer and teacher of creative writing as a self-therapeutic form of expression; she reviews expressive writing, especially poetry, as an alternative to the somatic management of essentially emotional problems. This section concludes with an exploration of perhaps the least acknowledged dimension of patients' experiences of themselves, their illnesses and the fount of their well-being, namely spirituality. Ilora Finlay, medical director of a Marie Curie Foundation hospice, reviews the ambiguity with which spiritual matters are handled in the existing medical and nursing literature and goes on to describe a study of the experiences expressed and reported by patients at a hospice day centre, as they come to terms with their own dying.

Again, let us preview these contributions in a little more detail. For Kieran Sweeney, the general practice consultation is a complicated and fluid experience, in which the doctor must balance research evidence, anecdotal experience, financial prudence, personal judgement and an understanding of the patient's narrative. In turn, the patient must also balance different considerations including their personal narrative and the actual or likely meaning of the problems which they are presenting to the doctor.

The consultation's central purpose is therefore the interpretation of the patient's story, involving perhaps a rather general subject matter described in words and images whose meaning may not be exactly shared by the participants. This is somewhat eased where there is long-term contact between a family doctor and a patient in a relationship of what Sweeney describes as solidarity and "compassionate witness". A doctor in such a relationship can, and should, avoid presuming that disease-free longevity is necessarily always the patient's goal. Doctor and patient exchange stories in metaphors that may reflect contrasting views of the world – and different types of knowledge. Medicine's current culture is one of evidence, but evidence is less straightforward in application to general practice than to specialist consultations. The dialogue adds a layer of nuance and interpretation to the supposed free-standing meaning of the evidence.

Sweeney also considers perhaps the most vivid experiential aspect of the consultation: the medical physical examination is a unique feature among professional relationships and the point at which the doctor exerts greatest power over the patient. A diagnosis following physical examination may condemn the person to the status of patient or, conversely, may bring the person back to normality from unfounded fear. Intimate bodily contact must not be allowed by sheer routine to be ignored for what it is – an invasion of personhood. The intimate physical examination proceeds from trust and respect between patient and practitioner or its dignity is lost – as is the patient's. Respect and trust must remain hard-earned and the dignity of the role must not be forgotten: even the "laying on of hands", Sweeney reminds us, is contact with the patient's *self*.

The very identity of self is at stake in our genetic constitution. Deborah Kirklin explores "the human backdrop" to the revolution in medical genetics and how the medical humanities might help to locate new technology and our understanding of it in the context of families" own narratives, our cultural and linguistic assumptions and our awareness of relevant historical developments – in short, our attempts to tell the stories of "what it means to be human".

Medical genetics and the new technologies of reproduction epitomise the impact of biotechnology on our self-understanding, argues Kirklin. Predictive genetic testing purports to offer us self-knowledge that can be both liberating (in offering choices) and constraining (in restricting the possibilities amongst which we can choose), as antenatal screening demonstrates when abortion is its principal "therapeutic" response to testing positive.

Scientific understanding has to be accommodated, received and interpreted alongside other candidates for the role of "theory", including those lay and folk explanations (often internally consistent) which may be constructed among families and other social groups. Kirklin considers as an example the "preselection" of individual members of at-risk families to be identified, often wrongly, as the sole bearers of the threatened condition. Another example is the wide variety of subjective perceptions and experiences of risk and, hence, of the impact of probabilistic genetic testing.

Moreover, the presentation of scientific results and implications is, for Kirklin, qualified by the choice of language used – as when discussion of genetic choices and interventions is "resonant" with the language of eugenics and of the often-clouded history which accompanies it. Understanding this history is crucial to understanding the language in which scientific development will be received, particularly when debates are sustained in, and shaped by, the mass media. Kirklin reflects upon the cloning debate and on embryo research in this connection and on the way that the choice of descriptions by a given discussant betrays the preassumptions (or "pro-attitudes") which he or she holds concerning the phenomenon in question.

Kirklin's conclusion is that biotechnological information is understood not in a vacuum but in the context of existing historical and family-contextual knowledge, lore, and belief. As such, it is incorporated into our re-telling of stories about ourselves; Kirklin sees the medical humanities as helping us to understand this, by "giving a voice to the many and varied perspectives involved".

One of the most intense contacts between "selves" in this sense can be found in the communication of thought and experience through expressive writing, perhaps most particularly the writing of poetry. Gillie Bolton professionally practises and teaches, and here reviews, the therapeutic potential of interpreting and communicating experience through such writing. She begins her discussion by asking how we could prevent grief, anxiety, and depression from becoming somatised as physical pain and distress. Such somatisation, she observes, often reflects a lack of emotional outlets for the patient. It is then reasonable to try to provide such outlets and helping people to express themselves in creative writing offers a potential therapy, though one that is not available within somatic medicine as such.

Poetry in particular is a succinct verbal exploration of deep and intimate thoughts and experiences and it can concern itself with the root causes and the felt "mode" of much emotional and even somatic suffering. Writing poetry can be compelling, absorbing and, argues Bolton, a source of self-confidence as well as providing an unusual vehicle for exploring difficult decisions. It is a highly deliberate process, contrasted with ordinary talking, and resembling a "dialogue with oneself". For Bolton, writing is also in its way more *physical* than talking and far less trammelled by the conventional expectations of verbal communication.

Bolton charts different stages of writing poetry: exploratory drafting can be followed by the discipline of redrafting and by the grammatical refinements of editing; all can be therapeutic. Making a somewhat controversial distinction, she urges that form in poetry serves to increase the impact of its content. The unformed, uncrafted material in a first draft can communicate powerfully (to others or to oneself) because of the experience which it conveys. Indeed, she suggests, poetry is more about journeying than about arriving and every turning is a surprise. Bolton points to evidence supporting the therapeutic properties of creative writing for the alleviation of somatic symptoms. Learning to live with oneself either in health or in sickness is not inherently easy. In attempting to do so, private creative writing – and supported reflection on that writing – offers us insight and guidance.

There is perhaps a fine line to be drawn between those intensely personal thoughts and feelings which might find expression in poetry and the experiences, attitudes, and beliefs which form our spiritual dimension. These too are important, though, as Ilora Finlay argues, also too little acknowledged in medicine and healthcare. For Finlay, "healthcare" actually deals in the business of managing illness and suffering rather than health as such and, as other contributors affirm, an important dimension of this concerns the emotional impact of suffering. The hospice movement has historically tried to respond to this impact, but a further dimension of patients' needs has emerged as a factor in their distress – their spiritual needs.

The extant literature deals only ambiguously with spiritual needs, in which specific religious ideas have become entangled, sometimes inappropriately and hence confusingly. Changing cultural norms have led to changes in the way that spirituality is discussed, such that for instance it now engenders the kind of embarrassment once reserved for public discussion of sexuality. The Christian basis of the hospice tradition in western care gives rise to difficulties with regard to spirituality grounded in other faiths or in no specific religious faith. Finlay reminds us that since spiritual needs are not quantifiable, they are not well handled by the modern emphasis on measurement in healthcare. Moreover, spirituality is an aspect of many relationships, of which a relationship with God is only one kind and one which is not present for everyone. In a modern secular society, spirituality itself can take a more secular form. Despite these complexities, finding appropriate responses to patients' spiritual needs forms an integral part of helping them in their search for meaning in their suffering.

With these difficulties in mind, Finlay reviews a study of patients' perspectives of pastoral, spiritual, and religious needs in a regional palliative care centre and how patients felt these needs were best met. The study, concerning patients from relatively impoverished post-industrial communities and using focus group methods with semi-structured discussions, disclosed a number of factors important in these patients' experiences and needs. These included the influence of previous bereavements; the difficulty of defining "spirituality"; the importance of humour in communicating difficult messages; the importance of a common bond between patients facing comparable illnesses and prognoses; loneliness or adversity in relationships generated through the stigmatising effects of terminal illness; the role of ritual in preparing for death; and, significantly, important sources of hope outside the formal institutional relationships between patients and staff. Finlay notes that these patients sometimes regarded clinical staff as being too busy to engage themselves in discussion of spiritual matters; she observes also that formal "counsellors" were frequently rejected as an avenue for therapeutic exploration. However, as she notes, the overall experience of day care attendance was highly valued as a context in which patients had had the opportunity to come to terms with their illnesses, offering as it did a context for connectedness and community (such as in the singing of well-loved hymns and secular songs) and for being listened to supportively.

Finlay concludes that the expression of narrative, and its being listened to, and a sense of wonderment at created life together constitute an essential part of being human, yet something not measurable in scientific terms.

At death's approach such aspects of the human spirit become more important than ever. No less than at other stages of life – indeed perhaps here more intensively than ever – the recording and interpretation of experience should be a compelling feature of the therapeutic relationship and the relevance of the humanities to clinical medical practice should be transparent.

# 5

# The consultation as Rubik's cube

Kieran Sweeney

Historically, the consultation has been analysed either strategically or semantically.[1-3] Both approaches have merit. The key contribution of the former was to ensure points of consensus between the patient and the doctor about the presenting problem and a potential solution to it. Pendleton and Hasler,[4] taking the latter approach, analysed the consultation innovatively and systematically, reflecting on patients' and doctors" attributes, as well as stressing the importance of the patient's health beliefs and concerns prior to the consultation.

In this chapter we develop a fresh explanatory model of the consultation. We propose a model consisting of six interrelated components and we use the metaphor of a Rubik's cube to elicit the difficulty of aligning each component into a pleasing symmetry which satisfies the hopes and needs of both participants. Those of us who remember grappling with the cube in order to align each side into a perfect monochrome will recognise the infuriating and elusive nature of such a task. We represent the consultation in this way for two reasons. First, it reinforces the notion that the consultation is a complex, fluid and dynamic dialogue: doctors balance new research against experience, they weigh clinical evidence against financial prudence, they measure the acceptability of their advice within the unique context of the patient's life.

And so do patients: they weigh up medical advice (and the precise manner in which it is conveyed) and place it within their personal narrative.

Second, this model allows us to dissect out each component of the dialogue, to show how both participants bring a series of different and sometimes conflicting paradigms to the consultation. Why do doctors think as they do? What are the beliefs underpinning the scientific knowledge which doctors use? How do patients come to act on advice about health? This model opens up these questions and explores how they relate to the decisions that emerge during the process. We conclude that the consultation is a dialectic, in which contributions from both parties are reciprocal, such that the outcome represents a (sometimes uneasy) compromise of the competing components.

The six components are shown in the box.

---

**The consultation as Rubik's cube: six components**

• The consultation as a forum for narrative
• The consultation as a forum for biomedical advice
• The consultation as a forum for disingenuousness
• The consultation as a forum for rationing
• The consultation as a forum for physical contact
• The consultation as a forum for acting a philosophy

---

## The consultation as a forum for narrative

Interpreting the patient's story is the central task of the consultation and transcends all others. The consultation in general practice is a dignified dialogue where the sick person tells a story to the professional advisor who in turn receives, evaluates, and interprets the story. This idea of the consultation as a forum for story telling introduces four key attributes of the consultation. These are the generality of the material, the process of interpretation, the linguistic building blocks of the dialogue and finally the dialogue as a dialectic.

Heath's definition of what she called the "mystery" of general practice is bound up with the concept of story telling.[5] Patients come to consultations with stories about anything: any issue, which an individual perceives as problematic and introduces into a consultation, becomes the legitimate business for the doctor. Recognition of the personal significance of an individual's story by another human being who understands its unique context is regarded by many as a prerequisite of the good consultation.[6-8]

Heath[5] argues that doctors have three key tasks: to interpret a person's story, to guard at the interface between health and disease and to witness an individual's suffering. Here, the word *witnessing* is used in a semi-biblical sense, to indicate the role of the practitioner as the recorder of events. The American physician anthropologist Howard Brody[7] asserts that a doctor acts as a fellow human being who has shared key events with an individual and, more importantly recognises their unique significance for that person. By doing this, the doctor helps that person make some sense of them. Knowing a patient perhaps for several decades, the doctor can witness the suffering, the struggle and the fortitude of the patient faced with a chronic condition that may be ameliorated, but never cured. The relationship, Heath argues,[5] is one of solidarity. Toon,[9] referring to this as the hermeneutic role of the practitioner, supports the view that doctors do not just intervene with biomedical weapons to ameliorate symptoms. The doctor participates in the consultation as a partner in the patient's struggle to come to understand illness and this is not merely a rational understanding but an understanding that involves emotions and contributes to the growth of the individual. General practitioners, educated as they are in the biomechanical model of curative interventionist care, are faced with a predicament. As their experience of practice matures, they find themselves inhabiting a world where the limitations of the biomechanical approach are increasingly exposed. Half of what they see cannot be diagnosed and three quarters of the conditions with which patients present cannot be cured.[10]

Conventionally, medical practice is predicated on the assumption that disease-free longevity is desirable. But it would be a mistake to presume that all patients share this approach. Skrabenek, in his classic text *The Death of Humane Medicine*, lamented this assumption.[11] He said that when the medical profession began to value longevity over intensity in the experience of living, it began to lose touch with the art of dying. Groucho Marx agreed with him. "The medics can now stretch your life out an additional dozen years," he commented, "but they don't tell you that most of those years are going to be spent flat on your back while some ghoul with thick glasses and a matted skull peers at you through a machine that's hot out of Space Patrol".[12] In *The Utility of Religion*, John Stuart Mill comments, "It is not naturally and generally the happy who are most anxious either for the prolongation of the present life or for a life here after; it is generally those who have never been happy". Witnessing, in the sense of participating in the compassionate care of an individual for whom biomedical interventions are increasingly ineffective, is at the same time one of the physician's central responsibilities and unique privileges. It may be unwise to presume that disease-free longevity is a shared and universal goal.

Seeing the consultation as a narrative helps us focus on the importance of the precise use of language by both the sick person and the doctor. "The words our patients speak to us are the closest we can come to the human experience of illness," Iona Heath argues.[13] "They represent only a shadow of the totality of that experience, but they express the most that we are able through language to share." The essential building blocks for any story are metaphors, themselves constructed from carefully selected words. Metaphors are one way in which we come to understand the world and they in turn reflect the type of knowledge we use to inform our actions. In any dialogue, the use of metaphor is central. Johnson and Lakoff's seminal text *Metaphors We Live By* contributes this thought: "Individuals draw heavily on metaphorical constructs in order to create meaning and to understand the nature of events. Without metaphorically based schemata the individual lacks an internal logic which allows for an understanding of the world. Reasoning based upon such metaphors is neither arbitrary nor unstructured".[14]

Some evidence is emerging that patients and doctors do not use the same metaphors when discussing a shared clinical problem and that this difference may contribute to a lack of congruence in relation to the problem.[15] And, as language reflects one's thinking, this linguistic difference may actually represent different types of knowledge that each participant brings to the consultation. For example, Piaget distinguishes between operational and figurative knowledge.[16] The former, which deals with logical connections and theoretical perspectives, is the preferred knowledge of professional groups. Figurative knowledge, on the other hand is the type of knowledge we pick up directly from everyday experience. Some recent work looking at how doctors and patients describe asthma suggests that they may understand the disease from differing epistemological standpoints. (K Edwards, personal communication)

The salient point for this model is that language is the currency of understanding; our use of language reflects the way in which we know things and make sense of the world. In the same way that doctors should not presume a shared philosophy of life with their patients, they must be aware of the potential for language to ensure transparency as well as create obfuscation. The precise choice of words is central to the flavour of the patient's narrative but no less important are the words chosen by the doctor to deliver advice.

# The consultation as a forum for evaluating and providing biomedical advice

Doctors in the National Health Service have a key responsibility to act as resources providing sound medical advice for patients who present with diagnosable medical conditions. To this end, the development of evidence-based medicine (EBM) has been central in creating an environment where practitioners and indeed patients are encouraged to clarify the basic clinical question in a presentation and to search for and appraise the evidence (where it exists) to answer it. Implementing such evidence and auditing the whole process completes the cycle of enquiry.[17, 18] EBM is now the new deity in medicine, espoused by clinicians, worshipped by managers and encouraged by politicians. An entire culture has grown up around the model.[19] Clearly no healthcare professional can abrogate responsibility for this: where the presenting complaint is clear and where there is evidence of benefit from a particular clinical response, there can really be no excuse for failure to act according to this model.

But the strong appeal of the EBM model is often not quite so straightforward to apply in the fluid and elusive forum of the primary care consultation. Critics of EBM have three main concerns. These relate to the nature of biomedical evidence, the way such evidence is evaluated, and the assumptions about implementing the evidence.[20]

For biomedical clinicians, the relative importance of evidence used in clinical consultations has up to now been clarified by two conventional layers of significance, statistical and clinical. Statistical significance is simply the mathematical likelihood that a result did not occur by chance. It is an agreed convention, which clarifies new medical evidence at the research level. However, its intrinsic weakness is the inevitably dichotomous nature of the evidence which it produces; things either are significant or they're not. Recent attempts by editors to encourage the use of confidence intervals have to some extent compensated for this, but they are equally reliant on a conventional understanding of probability derived historically by Sir Ronald Fisher at the 5% level. Clinical significance is an important additional factor which helps our interpretation of research findings at the level of regions, districts or practice populations. The consultation, however, is a one-to-one dialogue and another layer of significance is required to acknowledge the exchange of messages between the doctor and the patient.

Personal significance[21] adds a further dimension and is the key to the transfer of an idea too, and in the evaluation and interpretation of an idea by both the doctor and the patient together. Personal significance is thus dialectic. There are contributions from the practitioner, who offers an opinion, and from the person (patient), who receives and evaluates the new idea. Personal significance assumes that the relationship between the doctor and patient is horizontal, which sits uneasily with the conventional view of a hierarchical doctor–patient relationship.

Sweeney et al.[21] have argued that doctors carry out a dual evaluation of new medical evidence, based not simply on a mathematical clarification but on both a cognitive and intuitive evaluation of the material. There are three components to this evaluation: clarification of the evidence, followed by composition and transmission of the clinical message.

Patients are not simply passive recipients of these messages. They receive and evaluate them using cognitive and intuitive processes based on their prior factual understanding of the potential nature of a medical problem and their cultural, political, and social context. Thus although the consultation is a central opportunity for patients to receive biomedical information, any model which represents the implementation process as one-way traffic oversimplifies the nature of the event. This analysis illustrates how doctors and patients process this evidence and how that processing can affect the outcome of the dialogue and, more importantly, actions based upon it.

The relative contributions of the cognitive and intuitive components in a consultation will vary, depending on the context. In life-threatening situations, the cognitive component is likely to prevail. But in chronic disease or where therapeutic options are multiple, the balance of the two is likely to be much finer and, of course, different participants may attach different weights to them.

## The consultation as a forum for disingenuousness

To be disingenuous means to be lacking in openness, frankness or candour. In this section we argue that doctors have the potential to be disingenuous in four ways: about the philosophical assumptions which underpin their thinking; in assuming that consultations are value-neutral dialogues; in assuming they can rely on biomedical evidence to create clarity and certainty out of confusion; and finally in failing to recognise society's increasing scepticism about the biomedical model.

Contemporary medical practice is based on a "common-sense" view of science which regards scientific evidence as real because we can hear, see, and touch it. It is real, provable information, goes the argument, vigorously evaluated. But this principle rests on a circular argument and is deeply flawed.

The common-sense view of science in medicine is based on the principle of induction in which evidence is created by consistent serial observations. The *process* of induction, the argument goes, has proved satisfactory in circumstances a, b, c, ... so the *principle* of induction holds. Chalmers[22] elegantly demonstrates the flaw in this argument: it uses induction to prove induction.

In fact, most medical problem solving does not work in this way: the evidence suggests that doctors make decisions by constantly guessing and testing – using hypothetico-deductive reasoning, to give it its proper title.[1, 23] Others go further, arguing that general practitioners in particular act on hunches, seductively described as intuitive deductive thinking.[24] We argue here that in the consultation doctors can be disingenuous about their thinking, pretending that it is objective and robust.

In consultations doctors can also be disingenuous about the role of the self, particularly the doctor as self. The orthodox view is that consulting is an intellectually celibate activity, where doctors simply use objective scientific evidence to make decisions for patients. The evidence fails to support this view. Doctors are people too; they are not immunised by their medical education from holding personal attitudes, fears and views about health and disease. The fact that doctors are influenced by factors beyond firm science was first revealed by Bob Brook in his classic paper describing the work of British and American cardiothoracic surgeons.[25] He conducted an experiment in which cardiothoracic surgeons in the United States and the United Kingdom were exposed to an identical series of clinical vignettes and asked to evaluate the appropriateness of coronary artery bypass grafting (CABG) in each case. The surgeons in the US and the UK faced with the same clinical problems adopted quite different intervention strategies (the Americans advocated surgery more often). But how to explain this? Were not these doctors all part of the same profession, the same tradition, all positivists at heart? Brook was mystified: he ended his article by attributing the observed differences in clinical practice to "cultural differences difficult to quantify".

A comparison of prescribing in Europe five years later provided further evidence that cultural differences affected the way clinicians provided medications to their patients. Garattini and Garattini's *Lancet* paper in 1993 described the prescribing habits of doctors in four European countries, Great Britain, France, Germany, and Italy.[26] The researchers ranked the 50 most provided products in these countries into three categories as a function of the scientific evidence for their efficacy. In essence, their analysis showed that in the UK, the vast majority of products sold were supported by abundant evidence, while in France and Italy about half the products dispensed lacked any decent research evidence of efficacy. This report assumed, not unreasonably, that for the purposes of prescribing, European health professionals could be considered as a homogeneous community, as they supported the same biomedical paradigm, shared the same literature and increasingly exchanged its practitioners across its national boundaries. But if this was so, the implementation of their shared principles should have been more uniform. That it was not suggests that other, possibly cultural factors were operating.

For their part, patients are not just passive recipients of medical information, nor do they hold exclusively logical views on health. A person's attitude to health, and decisions about health matters, are determined by how that person perceives a particular threat to health, their belief in the advantages gained from a change in behaviour to accommodate the threat and how difficult that behaviour change is thought to be.[27] And the beliefs which form those attitudes to health are influenced by personal and family factors and by social and demographic factors.[28]

The recent spectacular rise of EBM as a model for clinical practice reveals another form of disingenuousness, this time about clinical certainty. The intrinsic appeal of the EBM model is that it holds out the promise of clarity. Most recently, the Secretary of State advocated "delivering the right evidence to the right person at the right time".[19] As a proposition this is virtually unknowable: it represents the subtle introduction of ideological language into health strategy documents. Clinical evidence is derived from population studies and *de facto* cannot predict with absolute certainty that a particular course of events will follow a medical intervention in a unique individual at any time. General practitioners along with their patients are faced with an almost unknowable heuresis through the illness experience. It is an unpredictable journey, influenced by many factors beyond the purely clinical.

Finally in the consultation doctors as a profession run the risk of being disingenuous about imposing medical strategies. Society is increasingly sceptical of the medical model.[29] Coercive healthism describes the predilection of the medical profession to go beyond educating and informing people about health. Skrabanek accuses doctors of resorting to propaganda to divide human activities into the approved and disapproved, healthy and unhealthy, prescribed and proscribed, responsible and irresponsible.[11] Will society continue to accept this? The last two decades of the 20th century have seen a gradual erosion of professional authority, particularly as a result of the well-publicised catastrophes in paediatric heart surgery and breast screening, as well as the Shipman case. The public's view of the medical profession has radically altered. The task for the profession is to construct a new way of relating to the public, based upon a much greater degree of transparency and collaboration.

## The consultation as a forum for rationing

The realisation that the National Health Service is unlikely to bear full responsibility for all the costs of sickness in society has been dramatically clarified by the introduction of dozenepil for dementia and sildenafil (Viagra) for impotence. The prevarication of the Secretary of State for Health, particularly over the latter, exposed the government's reluctance to fund new beneficial interventions regardless of costs. In comparison with other countries in the west, NHS funding is low – just less than 7% of the gross national product.[30] But there is no clear indication that increasing expenditure would result in any substantial improvement: the US healthcare system sustained by almost double that percentage of GNP, is still in considerable difficulty.[31]

Almost all the decisions a general practitioner makes have cost implications. They find themselves increasingly in paradoxical situations where careful clinical needs-based assessment leading to evidence-based prescribing can lead to unsustainable increments in prescribing costs. This brings them into increasing conflict with the newly formed primary care groups, which are driven by the politically sensitive principle of equity (Evans, personal communication). The inescapable fact is that general practitioners continuously make health economic decisions, balancing cost with cost alongside utilities, in effect trying to allocate quality of life values (ultimately a guess) to the evidence which may suggest benefits for the patient. But the principles of economics and the practice of medicine are uneasy bedfellows: market solutions based on a simplistic supply and demand model are simply not suitable.[32] The need for healthcare is uncertain and the information needed to make an appropriate choice between alternative strategies is not always readily available for the "consumer" (patient) to evaluate, and the concept of "utility", central to economic evaluations, is not a static given. Utility in this context refers to the satisfaction a person derives by consuming a product or making a choice between products. In health economics, the implicit assumption is that an individual will make a rational choice, maximising the utility derived from the resources available. But in a postmodern world, this assumption cannot safely be made: people (doctors included) are not always rational and choices between alternatives in clinical options will vary over time.

Thus, the practitioners are forced at times to make these choices on a patient's behalf, but as suppliers of care they cannot be seen as always impartial. Consider the general practitioner faced with a depressed patient and fully aware that her drug budget in the practice is substantially overspent. She may have to choose between antidepressants, which vary markedly in cost as well as therapeutic effect, or no drug therapy at all, relying on counselling as an alternative. How difficult is it to make those decisions impartially, with only clinical factors in mind? The fact is that decisions like these are taken daily in routine practice and are composed of an uneasy cocktail of clinical and health economic factors. These issues are likely to become more prominent as the National Institute of Clinical Excellence (NICE) begins to issue its guidelines for clinical care. It is likely to advise, for example, the lowering of cholesterol for patients with heart disease using medication the cost of which is unsustainable without either extra funding or a major redistribution of resources. The clinician is caught between a rock and a hard place, balancing the clinical imperative to identify patients with the condition against the economic imperative to reduce costs. Resources are scarce and every clinical decision carries its own option of opportunity costs. Sacrifice is inevitable.

## The consultation as a forum for physical contact

The physical examination sets the medical consultation apart from any other meeting between a lay and a professional person. It is one of the most important information-gathering behaviours associated with clinical practice and the part of the consultation when the doctor exerts the most power over the patient.[4] The very theatre of the clinical examination defines the power disparity between the participants: the doctor upright, fully dressed, and in familiar territory, with the patient lying prone, exposed literally and metaphorically. It can be a defining moment in which a person moves from the kingdom of the able-bodied to the paralysing uncertainty of the sick. Yet, despite its central importance in physical and emotional terms, relatively little has been written about it. Consider these two examples from the author's own experience. They are intended to illustrate two points about nakedness in the consultation: the connection between nakedness and loss of personal identity, and the huge privilege afforded to doctors who, unique among professionals, are permitted intimate access to a person's body.

Early in my medical training I attended the breast clinic of a prominent Scottish surgeon, during which women with suspected breast cancer were assessed for the first time. The patients were asked to undress in a side room before entering the consulting room where they faced not just the intimidating surgeon, but half a dozen young medical students too. The patients were usually offered a gaudy hospital towelling gown to wear. Early in the first clinic, an elegant woman, who appeared not to have undressed beforehand, entered the consulting room: she wore a black fur coat, fully buttoned up and offset by expensive jewellery. After a brief conversation the surgeon asked to examine the woman, who unbuttoned her coat, revealing that she was wearing nothing underneath. At that precise moment she symbolically left off her previous identity and entered the world of the patient, a role which a cursory physical examination of her breasts ensured she would never leave. The diagnosis of breast cancer, confirmed by the examination, had irrevocably altered the woman's status: she was now a sick person who would from that moment forward lose control of her destiny, surrendering it to medical people who, acting with the best of intentions, would forever consign her to a hierarchy in which she would be the subject.

Equally, the reassurance of a normal physical examination can bring a person back from the fear of sickness to normality. Consider the woman attending with a lump in her breast certain it is a cancer, only to find that the doctor's examination, followed by the removal of a small amount of cystic fluid, has completely removed the problem, physically and psychologically. Or the mother worried that her child's rash is a harbinger of meningitis, who gains huge relief from the reassurance of the doctor's assessment. The drama which accompanies the physical examination for the patient should not be underestimated, even in the most mundane clinical situations. For a sick person, the physical examination is the staging post between the worlds of wellness and illness.

For doctors the nature of the intimate bodily contact can become so routine that there is a danger of forgetting that each physical examination is an invasion of the individual's personhood.[6] Recently, at three o'clock in the morning, I attended a woman complaining of abdominal pain. I had never met her, nor her husband, but was immediately shown by him into the couple's bedroom, where the woman was obviously unwell. Within two or three minutes I formed the suspicion that she had an ectopic pregnancy. I asked her to allow me to perform a vaginal examination, which she permitted. Within the space of 10 minutes, I had met this woman, performed an intimate physical examination and summoned an ambulance in which she departed, leaving me in her own home with her concerned partner. No other person in society is given such privileged access to an individual's privacy: indeed for others, such actions would be criminal.

Virtually the only extended commentary in the medical literature on nakedness in medicine refers also to the sexual connotations inherent in the act of touching.[33] Sexual reactions to physical examinations are uncommon,[33] but always potentially present.[34] While doctors would regard most physical examinations as routine, this is not so for patients, who may react with a mixture of fear and embarrassment, particularly if ethnic factors influence the gender of the examiner.[35]

To address some of these concerns, the regular use of chaperones has been advocated in clinical practice, especially where that involves genital examination.[36] The evidence suggests that women, given the choice, would opt to have a chaperone present, while teenagers elect for a family member. The issue, interestingly, seems more contentious in specialist care rather than general practice where a substantial proportion of patients did not have a strong view on the matter in one study.[37] This may suggest that the trust and respect which emerge between a general practitioner and a patient form the catalyst which permits the intimate examination to proceed with dignity. But respect and trust are hard earned, are reciprocal and should never be assumed by the examining doctor.

Doctors are people too and may harbour their own reservations about clinical examinations in certain contexts and situations: some women doctors may feel less enthusiastic about performing rectal examinations readily on men and some male doctors an equal hesitation about vaginal assessment, for example in the patient's home. Homophobia may be just as prevalent amongst doctors as the wider population, with possible consequences for this part of the clinical assessment. The simple fact of having received a medical education does not excuse the profession for the normality of human prejudice: it may simply conceal it.

The principle for doctors is never to forget the dignity and sacredness of this role. It is a duty always to regard as a unique privilege the willingness of individuals to subject themselves to medical examinations. The very fact of laying on hands, even for the simplest of tasks like recording blood pressure, must always be seen as a contact with the person's interior self, a place where that person reigns unchallenged in times of health. And the potential for the physical examination to reclassify a person swiftly and dramatically as sick, with the attendant deconstruction of their intactness, should never be forgotten.

## The consultation as a forum for acting out a philosophy

Doctors are not great theorists but it is an inescapable fact that they act out a philosophy of medical practice every day. Historically, this philosophy emerged during the Enlightenment years. It has been heavily influenced by Francis Bacon's *Advancement of Learning*, in which the pathological findings in the morbid state were for the first time compared to the experience of being ill. Locke too was an important influence: his thinking underpins the scientific experiment which really constitutes the basic currency of scientific positivism. But above all, doctors are disciples of Descartes whose description of mind–body dualism remains a central tenet in medicine even now.

The Enlightenment produced a mechanical metaphor for the body. The body was machine: disease, an entity separate from the sick person, was simply a mechanical problem. Cartesian dualism, the positivism that derives from it and the rationalism which pervades clinical practice are testaments to the influence of this Enlightenment epistemology, which continues to dominate medical thought. Not everyone sees this as a worthy legacy. Evans and Sweeney have argued that the positivist approach actually represents an impediment to the central responsibility of doctors in any society – the relief of suffering.[38] The positivist approach to medicine has led to a celebration of abstracted decontextualised truths – truths emerging from scientific experiments in which the outcomes are distilled arithmetically. Such truths are abstracted from the context from which they arose – the unique story of the sick person – and as such can only ever be partial truths. And the linear notion of causality in the scientific experiment is criticised as being too simple to explain the constellation of influences which contribute to an illness experience.[38]

There is now a renewed interest in the importance of social and metaphysical risk factors for disease. Evidence is emerging of the influences of despair, hopelessness, and grief on disease. Reese and Lutkins published their seminal paper, "The mortality of bereavement", over 30 years ago.[39] Their finding of a seven-fold increase in mortality over one year in the relatives of a bereaved person indicated for the first time that death of a loved one carried a considerable increased risk of all-cause mortality in survivors.

Stress renders the immune system less competent.[40] Being poor, lacking control at work and feeling hopeless can all increase risk of coronary heart disease.[41] And Montgomery et al. were the first to show that family conflict could slow the rate of growth in children.[42]

In an important recent Occasional Paper from the Royal College of General Practitioners, Toon develops this issue by advocating a metaphysical basis for clinical practice.[43] He focuses on virtue ethics, describing courage, prudence, temperance, and justice as prerequisites of clinical practice. Justice, he argues, has to be the basis of all decisions of resource allocation. Both physical and moral courage are needed in consultations. Helping patients to maintain hope in the face of adversity and using compassion where all other biomedical interventions have failed are, in Toon's view, key roles of the general practitioner.

This is not an entirely new departure for doctors in the 20th century. It is rather a sign of them rejoining a centuries-old debate between the Aesclepian and Hygeian traditions in medicine.[44] In the former, health is seen as the absence of disease and the role of the doctor is to use external forces (treatment) to banish the disorder of disease. In the Hygeian model, health is regarded rather as a state of inner equilibrium: treatment is a way of restoring the physical, emotional, and spiritual elements of equilibrium, which have become unbalanced during illness.

Whichever tradition one prefers, whichever epistemological standpoint one adopts, the point is that the consultation is a forum for acting upon such fundamental assumptions. This analysis is not just an arcane or esoteric luxury; the epistemology of science is being denatured into an ideology in medicine: a political ideology to support government health policy and a professional ideology maintaining the role of the doctor in the health system. What is important is to make those epistemological assumptions explicit. Only then can they be evaluated.

## Conclusion

In this chapter we propose a model of the consultation based on six components which coexist in a fluid and unpredictable way. We have used the analogy of a Rubik's cube to represent the fluid nature of the dialogue (the sides moving one over another), the difficulty of reconciling the competing components (how infuriating are the attempts to achieve symmetry) and the vexed question of ownership (whose cube is it anyway? who decides when the cube is perfect?).

There is an enormous complex challenge inherent in every consultation. This is the central forum where a doctor conducts a dialogue with an individual who is autonomous, who may be frightened and who is at liberty to act on or ignore medical evidence in an unpredictable way. The model reveals the potential for disingenuousness: consulting is not an intellectually celibate activity. The model helps to explain the difficulties in translating what appears to be clear medical evidence into clinical practice. Impediments may exist either in the way evidence is evaluated by the doctor or in the transmission of clinical messages from the doctor to the patient. Sound medical advice may simply be ignored by the patients, no matter how robust the evidence is.

The model also invites the practitioner to reflect on the contradiction inherent in attempting to reconcile seeming opposites: science and art, uniqueness of the person and generalisability of the scientific experiment, the rights of the individual and those of society. Heath calls the product of these tricky combinations "uncertain clarity".[5] Far from torturing ourselves with the conflicts evoked by these dichotomies, Heath argues, we should revel in them. One of the spectacular achievements of biomedical science has been the extension of our knowledge of certain diseases by shifting the clinical focus from the particular, where it rested until the Enlightenment, to the general. The risk in this, however, is to devalue the fascinating uniqueness of every individual sick person. Isaiah Berlin recognised this distinction when he commented on Kant's philosophy: "Kant insists over and over again that what distinguishes man is his moral autonomy as against his physical heteronomy".[45]

The National Health Service is in a state of unprecedented change, the speed of which is bewildering. Its founding principles are confronted by political short termism, the language of its discourse threatened by the ideology of the elected. The physicist Nils Bohr is reported to have admonished a student for "just being logical all the time, not thinking". There is enormous pressure to do things in the health service just now: little opportunity and even less reward are afforded to those who feel the need to reflect, rather than act. This model provides food for such reflection.

# References and notes

1  Royal College of General Practitioners. *The Future General Practitioner: learning and teaching.* London: British Medical Association, 1972.
2  Roter DL. Patient participation in the provider patient interaction. *Health Educ Monograph* 1977; 5:281–315.
3  Stiles WB. Verbal response modes and dimensions of interpersonal roles: a method of discourse analysis. *J Personal Social Psychol* 1978; **36**: 693–703.
4  Pendleton D, Hasler J. *Doctor-Patient Communication.* London: Academic Press, 1983.
5  Heath I. *The Mystery of General Practice.* London: Nuffield Hospitals Provincial Trust, 1995.
6  Cassell E. *The Nature of Suffering and the Goals of Medicine.* Oxford: Oxford University Press, 1991.
7  Brody H. What does the primary care physician do that makes a difference? In: Stewart M (ed.). *Primary Care Research: traditional and innovative approaches.* Newbury Park, California: Sage Publications, 1991.
8  Dixon M, Sweeney KG, Pereira Gray DJ. The physician-healer: ancient magic or modern science? *Br J Gen Pract* 1999; **49**: 309–13.
9  Toon P. *What is Good General Practice?* Occasional Paper 65. Exeter: Royal College of General Practitioners, 1994.
10  Thomas KB. The temporary dependant patient. *BMJ* 1974; **1**: 59–61.
11  Skrabanek P. *The Death of Humane Medicine.* London: Social Affairs Unit, 1994.
12  Sherrin N. *The Oxford Dictionary of Humorous Quotations.* Oxford: Oxford University Press, 1995.
13  Heath I. Uncertain clarity: contradiction, meaning and hope. William Pickles Lecture. *Br J Gen Pract* 1999; **49**: 651–7.
14  Lakoff G, Johnson M. *Metaphors We Live By.* Chicago: University of Chicago Press, 1980.

15 Mabek CE, Olesen F. Metaphorically transmitted diseases: how do patients embody medical explanations? *Fam Pract* 1997; **14**: 271–8.

16 Piaget J. *Structuralism* (trans. C Maschler). New York: Harper and Row, 1970.

17 Sackett DL, Haynes RB, Tugwell P. *Clinical Epidemiology: a basic science for clinical medicine*. Boston: Little, Brown, 1985.

18 Sackett DL, Richardson WS, Rosenberg W, Haynes RB. *Evidence-based medicine. How to learn and teach EBM*. New York: Churchill Livingstone, 1997.

19 Secretary of State for Health. *A First Class Service*. London: Department of Health, 1998.

20 Sweeney KG. Evidence and uncertainty. In: Marinker M (ed.). *Sense and Sensibility in Health Care*. London: BMJ Books, 1996: 409–19.

21 Sweeney KG, MacAulay D, Pereira Gray DJ. Personal significance: the third dimension. *Lancet* 1998; **351**: 134–6.

22 Chalmers AF. *What is This Thing called Science?* St Lucia, Queensland: University of Queensland Press, 1978.

23 Marinker M. The Clinical Method. In: Cormach J, Marinker M, Morrell D (eds). *Teaching Clinical Method*. London: Kluwer Medical, 1981.

24 Willis J. *The Paradox of Progress*. Oxford: Radcliffe Medical Press, 1995.

25 Brook RH, Park RE, Winslow CM *et al*. Diagnosis and treatment of coronary disease: a comparison of doctors" attitudes in the USA and the UK. *Lancet* 1988; **i**:750–3.

26 Garattini S, Garattini L. Pharmaceutical prescriptions in four European countries. *Lancet* 1993; **342**: 1191–2.

27 Fishbein M, Azjen B. *Belief, Attitude, Intention and Behavior*. New York: Wiley, 1975.

28 Becker MH. The health belief model and the sick role behaviour. *Health Education Monograph* **2**: 409–19.

29 Le Fanu J. The fall of medicine. *Prospect* 1999; **July**: 28–31.

30 Office of Population Census Statistics, 1998.

31 Aaron H. *Serious and Unstable Condition*. Washington DC: Brookings Institute, 1991.

32 Kernick D, McDonald R. What is health economics and why do Primary Care Groups need to get to grips with it? In: Sweeney KG, Dixon M (eds). *The Emergence of Primary Care Groups: from rhetoric to reality*. Oxford: Radcliffe Medical Press, 2000.

33 Pereira Gray DJ. Nakedness in medicine. In: Pereira Gray DJ (ed.). *The Medical Manual*. Bristol: Wright, 1986: 146–53.

34 Jones RH. The use of chaperones by general practitioners. *J Roy Coll Gen Pract* 1983; **33**: 25–6.

35 Quereshi B. Muslim patients and the British general practitioner. In: Pereira Gray DJ (ed.). *The Medical Manual*. Bristol: Wright, 1986.

36 Bignell CJ. Chaperones for genital examination (editorial). *BMJ* 1999; **319**: 137–8.

37 Jones R. patients' attitudes to chaperones. *J Roy Coll Gen Pract* 1985; **35**: 192–3.

38 Evans M, Sweeney KG. *The Human Side of Medicine*. Occasional Paper 68. London: Royal College of General Practitioners, 1998.

39 Reese WD, Lutkins SG. The mortality of bereavement. *BMJ* 1967; **4**: 13–16.

40 Weiss JM, Sunder S. Effects of stress on cellular immune responses in animals. *Rev Psychiat* 1992; **11**: 145–80.

41 Brunner E, Davey Smith G, Marmot M *et al*. Childhood social circumstances and psycho social and behavioural factors as determinants of plasma fibrinogen. *Lancet* 1996; **347**: 1008–13.

42 Montgomery SM, Bartley MJ, Wilkinson RG. Family conflict and slow growth. *Arch Dis Child* 1997; **4**: 326–30.

43 Toon P. *Towards a Philosophy of General Practice: a study of the virtuous practitioner*. Occasional Paper 78. London: Royal College of General Practitioners, 1999.

44 Mitchell A, McCormack M. *The Therapeutic Relationship in Complementary Health Care*, London: Churchill Livingstone, 1998.
45 Berlin I. The apotheosis of the Romantic will. In: *The Crooked Timber of Humanity*. London: Fontana Press, 1991.

# 6

# The new genetics: retelling and reinterpreting an old story

Deborah Kirklin

Ah! These infantile sciences, these sciences in which one can only proceed timidly by hypothesis, and over which imagination still reigns supreme, they are assuredly the domain of poets quite as much as of *savants*. The poets go forward in the advance guard as pioneers, and often discover virgin lands, and point out the solutions which are near at hand. Between the acquired truths, those that are completely established, and the Unknown, whence the truth of to-morrow will be wrested, there is a space which fairly belongs to the poets. And what a huge fresco might be painted, what a colossal human comedy and tragedy might be written on heredity which is the very genesis of families and societies, of the world itself![1]

As Dr Pascal pours forth his vision of human heredity he echoes the claim made throughout this volume that the humanities could influence the very nature of medical understanding and endeavour. In this chapter I explore the human backdrop to the genetics revolution. This revolution will bring with it an intimate self-knowledge. As genetic understanding increases, the line between "us and them", "patients and public", will blur and perhaps disappear. Medical humanities offers a powerful way to help all of us – patients, healthcare professionals, and the public – to appreciate how the diagnosis of a genetic disorder impacts on those affected. Moreover, the humanities can help to contextualise this 21st-century lived experience within a cultural heritage rich in family lore. The history of genetics, marked by uses and abuses of knowledge of the mechanisms of heredity, both haunts and informs this field. An appreciation of the good and the bad ways in which man has, in the past, put this knowledge to use is essential if we are to understand the way in which our society responds to biotechnological advances at an individual and a policy level. This chapter will focus neither on the science of genetics nor exclusively on the associated ethical concerns although these will be mentioned from time to time. Instead the challenge facing man as he attempts to retell, reinterpret and add to existing stories about what it means to be human[2] will be examined.

## The new genetics

It is little more than 100 years since chromosomes were first glimpsed under the microscope and the importance of the deductive work of Mendel was finally appreciated. Since then developments have occurred at a remarkable rate and this year saw the realisation of one of the goals of the Human Genome Project when the entire human genome was decoded. This ambitious worldwide collaboration has allowed the genetically encrypted secrets of mankind to be revealed. Much has been discovered, much more remains mysterious.

It is now known that all human beings hold over 90% of their genetic code in common. The basis of over 4000 genetic disorders has been determined. Whilst cures for many of these remain elusive, there is increasingly widespread availability of the technology both for whole-population screening and for predictive screening of individuals known to be at risk of carrying specific genes. Thus it is now possible to screen individuals to ascertain whether they do in fact carry a genetic trait which might manifest itself as a disease and might be passed on to that person's children. It is possible to screen embryos before implantation into the mother's womb for specific genetic disorders and to implant only those free of the condition. It is even possible to select an embryo not just for the absence of a genetic trait but for the chance it offers of a cure to an already existing and affected sibling.[3]

When the "new" genetics is talked about there is a sense that it is not just the level of understanding that is considered new. The term "new" implies, to a lay audience, something conceptually novel. Beck argues that medicine has "created entirely new situations, has changed the relationships of humankind to itself, to disease, illness and death, indeed it has changed the world".[4] Beck's argument is not exclusively argued in relation to genetics but is argued also more broadly with respect to all of modern medical practice. Like all change, it is at the same time both exciting and frightening. The new reproductive technologies exemplify the conceptual challenges that have left society, sociologists, philosophers, psychologists, and politicians to ponder the impact of biotechnology on this relationship of mankind to itself. Egg, sperm, and embryo donation, surrogacy and, perhaps sooner rather than later, cloning have challenged the very meanings of mother, father, child, and family. As more and more individuals and families receive predictive information about their genetic load, concepts such as individual identity, confidentiality, and free will may lose their clarity and conviction. The "newness" or otherwise of the philosophical concerns raised by the new genetics has been addressed at length elsewhere.[5, 6] New or just more complicated, the questions raised are posed in particularly challenging ways. Foresight and imagination will be needed to address them. Patients, families, healthcare practitioners, philosophers, theologians, politicians, historians, and the public can all be expected to have views, hopes and fears for this rapidly expanding field of knowledge. The humanities can allow each one their say.

## Secrets and lies

There are secrets in all families.[7]

A devil, a devil born, on whose nature nurture can never stick.[8]

There is nothing new in the idea that we are born with certain characteristics. Indeed, when a child is welcomed into a family this is often accompanied by discussions of physical as well as temperamental resemblance to other family members. The idea that our roles in life are predestined as a consequence of these inherited traits is reflected throughout literature.[7, 8] In his epic Rougon-Macquart series, Émile Zola charts the occurrence of both moral traits and constitutional strengths and weaknesses throughout the family which gives its name to the series.[9] The family chronicler, Dr Pascal, sees his family history as holding a mirror to humanity:

...the history of our family, which is indeed the history of all families, the history of all humanity – much evil and much good.[10]

He passes on this "knowledge" about their family to his ward with trepidation but also with excitement and hope.

Perhaps the blow which the knowledge will deal you will make you the woman you ought to be.[11]

He recognises the dual-edged sword that (what we now call) genetic self-knowledge can be and this idea is echoed by numerous latter-day thinkers including the feminist Meg Stacey who says that "Knowledge may be constraining as well as liberating – sometimes both at once".[12] She is referring to the provision of choice (for example, to reproduce without the fear of giving birth to an affected child) and the restriction of choice (the loss of the ability to choose *not* to be informed about the opportunity for screening) that antenatal and prenatal screening can involve. The challenge for individuals and for society is to make a mature, measured and sustainable response to the freedoms provided by and constraints imposed by biotechnology during this coming of age. A grown-up approach is now needed if our humanity is to survive the unravelling of the human family's secrets and lies.

## Making sense out of uncertainty

Despite knowing there is "something in the family", not all families talk about their shared inheritance even when the members know the scientific basis of the disorder.

In our individual worlds I'm sure we all think about it, but as a family we never discuss it or bring these worlds together into one big world.[13]

When families do talk they often try to make sense of what happens within their family. Long before scientists explained about genes, families constructed their own explanations for the ways in which diseases affected them. These family theories have the trappings of internal consistency.

When I was young, my mother attributed her own breast cancer diagnosis to birth order. She talked about being the affected first-born daughter of an affected first-born daughter of an affected first-born daughter. She told me that as the first-born daughter in this line, I should expect to encounter the disease as well. With the diagnosis of one of my mother's younger sisters when I was twenty-five, my mother stopped talking about the disease as a problem of first-born daughters. Instead she dwelt on the personality traits that her affected sister shared with their mother – a certain intensity and vulnerability to stress looming large among them. Her focus implied that if a family history increased risk, it operated through some common temperament, either environmental or genetically shaped.[14]

This making sense can go further than explaining the past and can involve constructing a future for different family members according to the insights provided by the family's pseudo-scientific explanation of inheritance. Whilst sometimes this is done overtly and consciously, psychologists now recognise that it can occur subconsciously within families. An interesting example of how this can work is termed preselection.[15, 16] By singling out which family member will succumb to the family condition, the rest of the family are spared the pain associated with the uncertainty inherent in a late-onset disorder. Of course, in reality, they may find out, later on, that they have inherited the condition. Nevertheless, "knowing" they will not get the condition, they have not, up until this point of disillusionment, suffered the "have I, haven't I" anguish that not "knowing" entails. The following quotation from Martin Richards, writing in *The Troubled Helix*,[17] explains how this works.

> ...The process of pre-selection is unconscious and the individual selected may not be fully aware of what is being done. ...the process serves to reduce anxiety, and the non-selected individuals may say that they "know" they will not get the condition... the selected individual may speak of *when* they will develop the condition rather than if they will. .... (but, of course) families may get it wrong.

Preselection is just one example of how family scripts serve to define and order families" interrelationships.

> ...family relationships are not created *de novo* by each new

family member but there are beliefs about roles, relationships and individual characteristics that precede them and may help to produce their identity and place within the family. Such beliefs may be particularly powerful when a family is burdened by a serious genetic condition.[15]

If this is true then it must surely affect the way in which a scientific explanation about the individual risk status of members of the family is received and interpreted not only by the particular individual but also by the rest of the family.

## Screening, risk perception, and impartial advice

The new genetics promises to provide all of us with a lot of information about ourselves. Population screening seeks to identify individuals who might be at risk of either developing or passing on a genetic condition. Predictive testing seeks to determine whether or not a given individual possesses a specific faulty gene. Geneticists and genetics counsellors must explain these risks to people with varying levels of scientific understanding but even with a genetically literate audience, attempts at accurate risk communication can be frustrating. One of the reasons that families can find concepts of risk difficult to grasp has to do with the way in which people experience (rather than rationalise) risk.

> Each pregnancy, like a game of Russian roulette, is a gamble ultimately between life and death. For parents such as ourselves whose lives have been torn apart by a genetically inherited terminal illness, the risk factor so carefully calculated may be 1 in 4 or 1 in 24, but as we hold our breath with fingers crossed and wait for the results of yet another prenatal test, the odds will always be the same. An equal 50:50 chance. Why? Because at the end of the day the only results that really matter are either "it is" or "it isn't".[18]

Deciding whether to have a test, to find out whether you have inherited a genetic trait or not, must surely take great courage. Not surprisingly, counselling is considered an essential prerequisite and, in the tradition begun by John Fraser Roberts when he established the first clinic to offer genetic advice in terms of risk,[19] is non-directive. Despite rigorous attempts to provide information but not suggest one decision as preferable to any other, patient narratives flag up potential difficulties. The following observation by a woman with sickle cell disease, which amongst other things can make pregnancy and childbirth hazardous, reminds us that non-directive counselling can be inadvertently dominated by the standards for "normal behaviour" of the dominant group in society. Here it would appear that it was assumed by those providing counselling that an appreciation of the risk entailed in pregnancy automatically rules out having children as an option for the individuals involved.

> Undoubtedly many of us will die as a result of our pregnancies but many more will become mothers. While the risks have to be clearly spelt out, so too have success rates. We must be allowed to make our own choices.[20]

Another woman discusses the way in which she wished to receive the results of screening to see if she had inherited the gene for Huntington's disease. If she had inherited the gene, this would have foretold a premature, painful and humiliating death. The manner of her being given the result was very important to her. Her requests, although a deviation from normal procedure, would not have endangered her or markedly inconvenienced the medical team but were nevertheless refused. Her words serve as a challenge to the way in which all healthcare delivery is organised.

> Good or bad, this is how I wanted it. I remember saying perhaps they could treat each person as an individual and meet them half-way with this; after all, what works with one doesn't always work with another. Thankfully we are all different.[13]

Even within systems constructed with ostensible patient centredness and with non-directive counselling underpinning service delivery, it can appear to patients that feelings, as opposed to facts, are given little space.

> I still feel that many of the doctors and consultants I have met . . . do not appreciate the inner feelings I have; they have all been very matter of fact and give little opening for discussions of "feelings". They are much more willing to talk of physical health.[21]

If they are to rise to the challenge in these accounts then first of all doctors must be willing to face the shared pain that acknowledging the patient's and their own feelings will entail. Second they must understand that despite scientific explanations of risk, people's experience of risk often remains an "all or nothing" phenomenon. This knowledge must be accommodated in the practitioner's approach to explaining risk and to accepting choices that deviate from those they were anticipating.

## Choosing to know – or not to know

Receiving the results of predictive genetic testing can be an overwhelming experience even if the result is a good one. Here a negative result (the narrator has not inherited the Huntington's gene) brings mixed feelings and concerns about untested siblings. Again the lay perception of risk is evident.

> I feel such a huge sense of guilt, happiness, relief and isolation all mixed up together. Guilt because I was the lucky one. I've got no children to pass it on to, why me? What makes me different? I'm no better than them. Also sod's law says that one in three has a good chance of getting it, and I feel that I've narrowed their chances... [13]

The initial high of a good result is followed by a devastating low 10 days later.

> As high as these spirits were, they soon came crashing down on top of me. The same force which put me up there in my ivory tower pushed me deep into a big black hole, so big I felt I would never get out of it. ...I can only describe it as if someone is pushing you down with their hands on your head and shoulders. [13]

Not everyone decides to know. How do we as a society respond to people who prefer to play Russian roulette, who decide to shut their eyes, hold their breath, cross their fingers and jump in the deep end? The decision to do just that is often accompanied by guilt and a sense of stigma. One woman describes how she feels about having had four pregnancies in the full knowledge that she risked passing on the gene for Huntington's disease. She had not been tested herself but has an affected parent and therefore a one in two chance that she carries the gene.

I am aware that many people consider having a family of four a little excessive, perhaps somewhat inappropriate in today's world, maybe even irresponsible. I am therefore doubly aware that many people would judge having four children when at risk of a genetic disease to be the height of irresponsibility. I certainly cannot justify having four children myself, nor do I have any great expectation of others" understanding this choice. All I can say is that despite having had three children I still longed for more, and particularly, having three sons, I longed for a daughter. In these circumstances, it somehow seemed acceptable for us to impetuously "try" for a baby on just one or two occasions – and somewhat surprisingly, the result was our daughter.

... I have never felt there was anything to be gained by seeing a genetic counsellor. Perhaps I have also assumed that most people, including genetic counsellors, would feel some criticism of the choice to have children when at risk of having a genetic disease, and have no wish to be judged in this way. Indeed it is the reason why, since telling one or two friends when I was in my teens, I have avoided telling any friends, or indeed my partner's family, about the disease.[22]

Is she correct? Does society judge those who play Russian roulette? Does this judging enter into the non-directive encounter between genetic counsellor and client? It has been pointed out before that the very way in which we assess the success or failure of screening programmes, by measuring the reduction in the number of affected births,[23] precludes the possibility that a valid course of action after adequate counselling is to proceed with an affected birth. This may help explain the perception that refusal of screening or a decision not to let known risk status influence reproductive behaviour runs counter to what the medical team and society consider appropriate.

## History: lessons and legacies

The happiest women, like the happiest nations, have no history.[24]

In George Eliot's day women not only had to ensure that they had no history (or to hide what they had) but, as in her case, sometimes went to extraordinary lengths to conceal their very womanhood in order to succeed in the male-dominated world of the day. Nowadays many women will have a rich and colourful history before, and indeed if, they ever settle down to motherhood and family life. The life experience they bring to the family is arguably one of its great strengths.

Perhaps, as with women, so with nations and their histories. Since George Eliot's day the histories of the colonial powers, which at that time rode high in glorified self-esteem, have, with the perspective of time, become less a source of national pride and more a cause of collective reflection and self-doubt. Modern warfare, genocide, and the brutality of civil conflict have left numerous nations and their peoples burdened with a history bearing testimony to man's inhumanity to man.[25] Some of this history involves evil perpetrated in the name of eugenics with individuals sacrificed in the name of the greater good of "society". Much of the evil done was predicated on a presumption of the superiority of one group of people over the other with science invoked as "proof" of this. An understanding of this history is important if we are to have any hope of learning from the past. I would argue that an historical understanding of why we feel such unease at certain biotechnical developments will add an important perspective and enable more considered public and professional decision making.

It is not my intention to try to summarise the history of eugenics. Many scholars have done this already.[26] What interests me for the purpose of this chapter are the echoes of this past in the day-to-day discussions of developments in human genetics. First I will describe the highly charged media furore that greeted the birth of baby Nash and draw tentative conclusions as to the influence of historical events on the way these events were portrayed. In the final part of this chapter I will suggest that an understanding of the way in which language is used in philosophical discourse about biotechnology is essential for a meaningful debate and that the humanities have an important role to play in facilitating that understanding.

## Bred or born?

Baby Nash was a very much wanted baby. His parents already have one child, born with a rare genetic disorder called Fanconi's anaemia. As part of this condition she had developed leukaemia and needed a stem cell transplant if she was not to die prematurely.

When the Nashes decided to have another child, preimplantation diagnosis offered the opportunity to screen all of their embryos so that only those free of the inherited condition would be implanted. This was not a new procedure. What was new was that doctors also screened the embryos to ensure that any baby born to the Nashes would also be a perfect stem cell donor for their first child, Molly. The rights and wrongs of baby Nash's birth are not my concern here. What is of interest here is the way in which the media portrayed the ethical issues concerned.

*The Times* newspaper headline read, "Baby bred to save sister". *The International Herald Tribune* led with a front-page story entitled "Baby's cells to aid sister". By coincidence, on that day I was facilitating a seminar with undergraduate medical students about the way in which the media portray advances in genetics. The group began by focusing on the headlines chosen by these two papers. The group was unanimous that the words "bred" and "aid" jumped off the pages. A word association game starting with each of these words in turn came up with *bred, animals, horses, food, use, abuse* and *aid, help, rescue, save, hope*. The idea of breeding humans was clearly distasteful to the group. They didn't relate the language used to eugenic ideas. Nevertheless they felt breeding babies was wrong and the journalistic message seemed, to them, loud and clear. The word "bred" and its suggestion of human husbandry has, for those familiar with the history of eugenics, a strong resonance with that movement. Francis Galton, the so-called father of eugenics, described his eugenic theory thus:

> Natural selection rests upon excessive production and wholesale destruction; Eugenics on bringing no more individuals into the world than can be properly cared for, and only of the best stock.[27]

In America in 1904, Charles Davenport established a station for the experimental study of evolution. Davenport was attracted to Galton's emphasis on the procreation of good stock and compared a woman's choice of a spouse to the stockbreeder's choice of "a sire for his colts or calves".[28] I would hazard that the students' reactions to the news coverage were echoed throughout the country as people read *The Times*" headline. Distrust, distaste, discomfort. These students read on, understood the science, had seen what leukaemia can do to a child, and judged for themselves. Is that true for most people? How much are the public, or for that matter the journalists and editors of our newspapers, conscious of the eugenic legacy that affects so fundamentally the reporting of developments in this field?

These concerns are echoed in the recurring public debates about designer babies, the idea that couples might use the new genetics to select or deselect babies for traits that are trivial, discriminatory, and demeaning. Even individuals who, like the students, do not consciously recognise the effect of the history of eugenics on their reactions to technological developments nevertheless react strongly against the language of eugenics. Whilst informed, to varying degrees, about the murders, sterilisations, and incarcerations that have taken and continue to take place in the name of eugenics, they had not thought of their reactions to the *The Times*" article as stemming from this knowledge.

Once this point was raised, an initial irritation with the inflammatory language used by the journalist gave way to a wide-ranging discussion of the concerns such technology might raise. I would argue that acknowledging the influence that the history of eugenics has had on our evaluation of current developments would at least bring these reservations and concerns to the debate. If mankind is to learn any lessons from history then let us examine that history consciously and openly with reminders about the eugenics of today and yesterday well signposted and not slipped, disingenuously, into media headlines. If (as I have suggested) there is indeed a "subtext" to media coverage, then, given the power of the media in influencing public debate and opinion, it should be revealed for all and not just the well informed.

Baby Nash has, it appears, been able to aid his sister. Surely every parent shares in the Nashes" joy. Open discussion of the historical perspective on this case would surely facilitate the analysis of whether it constitutes a use or misuse of science. Denial of the fears born of history could, on the contrary, lead to an entrenching of positions that would be unhelpful and potentially destructive.

## The power of language and the cloning debate

We have seen that words are important in reflecting and shaping attitudes. It is not my purpose here to revisit the ethical arguments about the rights and wrongs of cloning. I will focus instead on the language employed in the ongoing public and policy debate and suggest what this can reveal to the alert reader about the attitudes and agendas of those involved.

The unusual language employed in the public discussion of cloning provides an interesting example of this. In 1998, the Human Genetics Advisory Commission (HGAC) and the Human Fertilisation and Embryology Authority (HFEA) circulated a consultation document addressing the scientific, ethical, and social issues raised by human cloning.[29] The document was sent to a selected audience of concerned professionals and organisations representing scientific, legal, clinical and ethical interests. The document's authors decided to introduce novel terminology to distinguish between the different potential outcomes of applied human cloning technology.

> ... "human reproductive cloning", that is the production of genetically identical human beings, which is banned: and what may be broadly called "therapeutic cloning", which (although not coterminous with scientific usage) may be used to describe other applications of nuclear replacement technology, which do not involve the creation of genetically identical individuals.[29]

Given the history of IVF and embryo research, coupled with the media excitement that surrounded Dolly the cloned sheep, the careful use of language in the HGAC document is perfectly understandable. The *Boys from Brazil*[30] spectre is at once acknowledged by the reminder that such work is banned. Interestingly the term "non-therapeutic" was not used to describe this type of cloning. The description actually used – "human reproductive cloning" – seems to avoid a value judgement. Therapeutic cloning by contrast conjures up an image of benefit flowing to needy individuals. The creation of embryos using cloning techniques is integral to both and we should be clear that therapeutic cloning would involve extensive embryo research. This implication was quickly identified by a cross-section of the public canvassed at that time.[31] Moreover, these embryos will not be "spare" embryos arising out of a treatment programme but rather purpose-made.[32] Any failure to appreciate this might well be compounded by the reassuring statement that human reproductive cloning would involve the production of "genetically identical human beings", whilst therapeutic cloning would not produce "genetically identical individuals". Of course, if we accept the argument that until 14 days there is no "individual" and limit research using cloned embryos to 14 days then this would be a technically correct statement.[33]

Another consequence of the choice of language in this document has also been noted.

> By placing the emphasis on cloning and then distinguishing between reproductive and therapeutic purposes, the consultation document obscures an essential prior step: the creation of human embryos (cloned or otherwise) for research purposes beyond those permitted in the 1990 Act. Whether there is additional moral significance in the fact that the embryo might have been produced by nuclear substitution is a separate matter from the morality and legality of creating any embryo for purposes other than those permitted in the Act.[31]

The use of language in the consultation document, with its focus on ends rather than means, is, I would suggest, a reflection of the pro-research stance of the authors. The utility of this work appears to be the main evaluative tool being used by the authors. The means (creation of embryos for research) does not feature in their descriptive language and instead the benefits of this "therapeutic" work are implicit in the language employed. It is of interest to recall the language employed in the original heated debates, both public and parliamentary, that preceded the introduction of the Human Fertilisation and Embryology Act in 1990. This Act of Parliament allowed strictly regulated experimentation on human embryos up to 14 days after fertilisation for a limited number of purposes. At that time the term "therapeutic embryo research" was used to describe research that aimed directly to benefit the embryo that was the experimental subject. "Destructive research" was the term used to describe embryo research that would be of no value to the experimental subject itself and would end with its destruction. The power of language, carefully employed, is illustrated by considering how different "therapeutic cloning" sounds if re-described as "destructive cloned embryo research".

Naturally, the value that the authors place on the potential benefits of such technology will be shared by many of us concerned with this field. Nevertheless, pre-existing or pro-attitudes suggested by the use of language of the consultation document's authors is an instructive starting point when trying to understand why embryo research is an area where consensus often seems unattainable. For clarity's sake I will explain what I mean by pro-attitudes before analysing why identifying them can be helpful.

# Pro-attitudes

The term "pro-attitude" was first coined by Nowell-Smith in 1954.[34] It was subsequently adapted by Donald Evans and used to explore the relationship between how we describe the human embryo and how we choose to treat it. He explains:

> How we are prepared to act towards the embryo demonstrates our choice of how we shall describe it. That choice is impeccably explained by the *pro-attitudes* we hold towards the description of the embryo. In turn these *pro-attitudes* provide impeccable reasons for our describing the embryo as we do.[35]

Let us look again at the language used in the consultation document, bearing in mind Evans" explanation of pro-attitudes. Cloned embryo research is described as therapeutic. The choice of such language to describe this type of research implies a positive, accepting attitude towards such research. The implied approval of therapeutic cloning would explain any choice made in the future by such a group to sanction such research. So advice from the Authority (assuming that the majority views of the Authority members are reflected in the pro-attitudes we have inferred), to the Secretary of State, that he allow such research in the future could be seen as internally consistent with their own pro-attitudes. This is, of course, just one example of how pro-attitudes might colour the nature of the debate. Given that the different pro-attitudes held by individuals will affect so directly the language they use, what effect does this have on the nature of the debate surrounding the morality of human embryo research?

During the period since I first advanced this argument in 1998[36] the committee charged with advising the government on the conclusions of the above consultation exercise recommended that, whilst reproductive cloning should remain banned, therapeutic cloning should be allowed within strictly regulated guidelines.[37]

It is clear that the cloning debate involves a continuation of the personhood debate so familiar from discussions about the moral acceptability of abortion.[31] This is not a "new" point of contention but another version of a debate which can leave reasonable and intelligent individuals with little common ground. It is hardly surprising that those in favour of allowing cloned embryo research to go ahead (given the potential benefits to, amongst others, those affected by genetic disorders) did not want to open up the abortion debate again. Being in favour of this research myself I can sympathise with these concerns. I welcomed the Donaldson report and the conclusions it drew.[37] Nevertheless if such important issues are to be aired for public consultation then a clear and open appreciation of the starting point of all those involved is necessary to give the public confidence in the conclusions reached. The first in-depth analysis of public opinion, conducted by a research charity using qualitative methods, has shown that despite the language of the HFEA/HGAC consultation document, the lay public is quickly able to grasp the key moral issues associated with cloned embryo research. This analysis revealed that increasing "concern and apprehension" mirror any increase in the public's understanding of these scientific issues.[31] Despite this, and indeed because of this, consultation should move beyond "a selected audience of concerned professionals and organisations".[38] Zola's vision of the poet offering a perspective unavailable to the savant of science is perhaps too simplistic a portrayal of the relative merits of each. I would suggest rather that the range of insights and perspectives available to both would, when combined, result in a fuller understanding of what it is to be human.

# Conclusion

Don't let us forget that the motives of human actions are usually infinitely more complex and varied than we are apt to explain them afterwards, and can rarely be defined with certainty. It is sometimes much better for a writer to content himself with a simple narrative of events.[39]

The genetics revolution is not taking place in a scientific vacuum. Biotechnology will increasingly provide individuals and families with information that cannot be understood independently but will need to be added to and reconciled with existing family lore. Society will reach conclusions about the rights and wrongs of using technological skills not in isolation but within an historical context rich with important lessons for us all. Medical humanities, by giving a voice to the many and varied perspectives involved, can offer invaluable help in the retelling and reinterpreting of the complex human story that lies at the heart of the new genetics.

# References and notes

1   Zola E. *Dr Pascal*. Stroud: Alan Sutton Publishing, 1989: 113.
2   Numerous cultures have created stories to explain the origin of mankind. An example is provided by the Old Testament's *Genesis*. The importance of free will is emphasised in this story: man can choose to act for good or evil and these choices are available to all. However, with increasing knowledge of genetics the relationship between "nature" and "nurture" is once more under scrutiny. Questions such as "Can free will ever be exercised?" are being asked. For an analysis of these issues see, for instance, Radcliffe Richards J. *Human Nature after Darwin*. London: Routledge, 2000.
3   The "Nash case" as reported in *The Times* and *The International Herald Tribune* on October 9th 2000; details are discussed later in this chapter.
4   Beck U. *Risk Society: towards a new modernity* (trans. M Ritter). London: Sage, 1992.
5   Singer P (ed.). *Embryo Experimentation: ethical, legal and social implications*. Cambridge: Cambridge University Press, 1990.
6   Harris J. *The Value of Life*. London: Routledge and Kegan Paul, 1985: see Chapters 1 and 8.
7   Farquhar G. *The Beaux' Stratagem*. London: A and C Black, 1998: III, iii.
8   Shakespeare W. *The Tempest*: IV, i.
9   *Dr Pascal* is the final novel in the 21-volume Rougon-Macquart series which follows the fortunes of this family through the second empire in France. For Zola *Dr Pascal* is "a scientific work, the logical deduction and conclusion of all my preceding novels", in which he presents his ideas on the role of heredity in men's lives.
10  Zola[1], 108.
11  Zola[1], 109.
12  Stacey M. *Feminism*. In: Marteau T, Richards M (eds). *The Troubled Helix*. Cambridge: Cambridge University Press, 1996: 340.
13  Madigan J. Needing it like this. In: Marteau T, Richards M (eds). *The Troubled Helix*. Cambridge: Cambridge University Press, 1996: 7–26. Here she discusses her family's response to carrying the Huntington's gene which causes a premature, painful and terminal neurological disease in sufferers.
14  Macke E. A family history of breast and ovarian cancer. In: Marteau T, Richards M (eds). *The Troubled Helix*. Cambridge: Cambridge University Press, 1996: 32.
15  Kessler S. Invited essay on the psychological aspects of genetic counselling. V. Preselection: a family coping strategy in Huntington's disease. *Am J Med Genet* 1988;**31**: 617–21.
16  Kessler S, Bloch M. Social systems responses to Huntington's disease. *Fam Process* 1989; **28**: 59–68.
17  Richards M. Families. In: Marteau T, Richards M (eds). *The Troubled Helix*. Cambridge: Cambridge University Press, 1996: 269.
18  Hearnshaw H. A mother's account. In: Marteau T, Richards M (eds). *The Troubled Helix*. Cambridge: Cambridge University Press, 1996: 47. A mother discusses how she and her husband understood the risk of a second child being born with Wernig–Hoffman's syndrome, an inherited terminal neurological disease which their first child had already died of.
19  Roberts JAF. *An Introduction to Human Genetics*, 2nd edn. Oxford: Oxford University Press, 1959.
20  France-Dawson M. Some observations about my life with a sickle cell condition. In: Marteau T, Richards M (eds). *The Troubled Helix*. Cambridge: Cambridge University Press, 1996: 49.
21  Anonymous. An ordinary experience. In: Marteau T, Richards M (eds). *The Troubled Helix*. Cambridge: Cambridge University Press, 1996: 38. Writing from

the perspective of someone with a strong family history of breast and ovarian cancer.

22 Anonymous. Living with the threat of Huntington's disease. In: Marteau T, Richards M (eds). *The Troubled Helix*. Cambridge: Cambridge University Press, 1996: 24.

23 Modell B, Petrou M. Thalassaemia screening: ethics and practice. In: Cruikshank JK, Beevers DG (eds). *Ethnic Factors in Health and Disease*. London: Wright, 1989.

24 Eliot G. *The Mill on the Floss*. London: Blackwood, 1860: Chapter 3.

25 Glover J. *Humanity: a moral history of the twentieth century*. London: Jonathan Cape, 1999.

26 Kevles DJ. *In the Name of Eugenics: genetics and the uses of human heredity*. New York: Alfred A Knopf, 1985.

27 Galton F. *Memoirs of My Life*. London: Methuen, 1908.

28 Davenport C. *Heredity in Relation to Eugenics*. USA: Henry Holt, 1911: 248–9.

29 Human Genetics Advisory Commission. *Cloning Issues in Reproduction, Science and Medicine*. London: HGAC, 1998.

30 *The Boys from Brazil*, a 1970s Hollywood film, involves a group of Nazis, led by the notorious Dr Mengele, who clone a number of male babies from Adolf Hitler's tissue and then place them in families chosen to resemble Hitler's own.

31 The Wellcome Trust. *Response to the HGAC/HFEA Consultation on Cloning Issues in Reproduction, Science and Medicine*. London: Wellcome Trust, 1998.

32 It should not be, but often conveniently is, forgotten that current legislation already allows embryos to be created specifically for research. Here the eggs and sperm are donated for this purpose. Calling these embryos "spare" is misleading. Spare (as regards the HFEA legislation) means embryos *created with the intent of implanting them in the mother's womb*, but subsequently found not to be needed. Intentionally creating more embryos than are required for potential implantation, with or without the egg and sperm donors' permission, is a different matter. Such embryos are not "spare". They have been created specifically for research.

33 Not all accept the "no individual" argument; see, for instance: Evans M. Human individuation and moral justification. In: Evans D (ed.). *Conceiving the Embryo*. The Hague: Martinus Nijhoff, 1996: 75–85.

34 Nowell-Smith PH. *Ethics*. Harmondsworth: Penguin, 1954: 111–21.

35 Evans D. Pro-attitudes to pre-embryos. In: Evans D (ed.). *Conceiving the Embryo*. The Hague: Martinus Nijhoff, 1997.

36 Kirklin D. *Public consultation on human cloning begins: an opportunity to examine the role of pro-attitudes in the embryo research debate and their effect on legislation*. Thesis submitted as part of MA in Medical Ethics and Law, King's College, London, 1998.

37 Donaldson L. *Stem Cell Research: medical progress with responsibility*. London: Department of Health, 2000.

38 HGAC[29]. This phrase was included in the cover letter that accompanied the consultation document.

39 Dostoyevsky F. *The Idiot* (trans. D. Magarshack). Harmondsworth: Penguin Classics, 1955: 463.

# 7

# Poetry as a key for healthcare

Gillie Bolton

*The captain unlocked his word-hoard.*[1]

*Poetry is ampoules of the purest, clearest drug of all, the essence and distillation of the process of living itself.*[2]

*I would define medicine as the complete removal of the distress of the sick, the alleviation of the more violent diseases and the refusal to undertake to cure cases in which the disease has already won the master, knowing that everything is not possible to medicine.*[3]

Once upon a time a pilgrim asked where he might find his heart's desire. The wise woman studied him hard and long with wide-set emerald eyes before saying: "You have a long way to go and it will take a long time". He took her hand and kissed it, holding it for longer than he need. As he left, eyesight blurred with tears, she sped him on his way with: "You will know when you have found the right person, they will offer you their hat".

Our seeker after the Truth travelled over oceans, deserts, forests, mountains, and torrents, through weeks, years and decades. He became weather-worn, travel-wise, and weary but knew he was on the right trail. He came to a glade dappled with soft sunshine, carpeted with bluebells, stitchwort, and golden celandine. A woman got up as if expecting him and reached up to put her garland of wild-flowers on his head. "Now you can share my crown." It was the same woman he left so long before. And they lived happily ever after.

Gillie Bolton

However hard the search, however much energy and money expended, the solutions to life's biggest problems are usually right here and now, if only we can perceive them. When "the captain unlocked his word-hoard", all he did was speak.

How do we support people towards gaining the kind of strength necessary to bear the griefs, depressions, and anxieties they suffer? How do we prevent emotional and mental distress being expressed in physical pain? Henry Maudsley said of such somatisation: "The sorrow that has no vent in tears makes other organs weep".[4]

The thesis of this chapter is that helping people unlock their word-hoards in poetry can offer them a therapy not possible to medicine, or perhaps one additional to medicine and nursing as it is currently understood. Poetry can be powerful in the therapeutic search for acceptance of life's vicissitudes, peace of mind, and even joy. The process of writing and sharing that writing very often allows the tears to flow. This chapter offers some insight into why poetry writing has such impact, exemplified by the work of patients and clinicians.

## Poetry in particular, and writing in general

Poetry is an exploration of the deepest and most intimate experiences, thoughts, feelings, ideas: distilled, pared to succinctness, and made music to the ear by lyricism. Poetry often makes use of image, such as metaphor or simile, to express vital experiences in a few words.

Poetry writing is compulsive, utterly absorbing for these reasons, and therefore tends to be self-affirming and confidence enhancing, as well as challenging and demanding. The very creative process is enjoyable and rewarding. Poetry, as an art, is a gift to the self.

This is writing which expresses things from deep within, explores things people didn't know they knew, felt or remembered. It offers endlessly creative questions and tantalising paths to follow, rather than answers. It can also explore issues which are known about but difficult to sort out, such as a life decision "Shall I take that job?", or a problem at work.

Writing can do this partly because it is private. No-one watches and listens to every word; it need never be shown to anyone – possibly not even reread by the writer. The rereading of writings, and particularly the sharing of them with others, is a conscious, deliberate process, very different from talking.

Writing is a gentle and paced process of personal development – I have never known anyone write more from their inner self than they can cope with at that time. It is easier in writing than in speaking to stop in mid-phrase when it gets painful.

Polonius exhorted his son, Laertes: "To thine own self be true".[5] This always puzzled me: how does one find one's own self in order to be true to her(him)? I now feel that listening to the inner voices which dictate poetry is close to what might be a dialogue with my own selves, a search for integrity and wholeness despite the multiplicity. It is the search for "true" self-contact in a similar sense that a straight line is "true". I think Ann Kelley probably meant something similar:

> Poems are simply ways of telling the truth and distilling the truth of our emotions. We may think we are writing about a hobby or a memory, a dream or a garden, but something of the writer's "soul" comes out in the chosen words and speaks to the reader.[6]

## Poetry from the hospice

Muriel's poetry is an example of this. Muriel was an elderly cancer patient at a hospice. She participated in several workshops I set up in the dayroom and also worked with me one to one. Here is her first poem:

Everything seems like a ball of string
all tangled up, with crinkles in
as if it's been unknitted
that's just how I feel
it's neither going straight nor the other way

one night I said my prayers
and thought, will things ever sort themselves out?
first I think one way
and then I think the other.

I try to be brave
and look on the bright side
but it's one step forwards and one step back,
things are closing in on me
and it's all twisted up
I don't know.

Things keep cropping up
things happen that fast
I can't keep control of it.

> After Christmas
> after all this darkness
> I'll be able to go forwards
> things will lift.
>
> It'll be a newly rolled ball of string.

Muriel initially ended with "things will lift". She was delighted when I pointed out the development in her poem: from tangle to light. I asked her what the ball of string would be like in the New Year; she provided the last line.

Muriel's use of image is startlingly effective. Her simile "everything seems like a ball of string" is one I am sure we can all relate to, even if not struggling with cancer. This simile was satisfying to her: as though she was able to hang on to both ends of her string, secure in the knowledge that string is untangleable. The hope in this poem is tangible, despite the feeling of muddle.

Muriel wanted to write about a dream shortly afterwards, having taken more notice of dreams since our writing about them at a workshop. She gave some background: "I have a tortoise. I look after it in the winter. I put it in the bottom cupboard. I was dreaming about my tortoise, and I was still in the dream when I woke up."

> Outside it was deep in tortoises;
> little ones and big ones everywhere
> I've never seen such little ones,
> brown ones, green ones
> all sorts of tortoises
> I was digging them up
> out of the ground with my hands.
> They were lovely little tortoises
> and I saw one's little legs
> and they were green
> and I thought "fancy that".

Once more the use of image is graphic. What a sense of burgeoning life in this mass of green-legged tortoises, relating to the feeling of hope and light at the end of the first poem, rather than the dreariness of the tangle. These poems were written just before Christmas, a common time for dying or depression, along with January. Underneath Muriel's lowness, struggling with the effects of cancer as nearly all the patients were, was this bubbling of hope, reinforced by the writing of the poem. The hope was communicated to the other patients when they heard the poem.

## Poetry for the dying and the bereaved

Betty Roddie died aged 39 of breast cancer in 1974. Just before she died she wrote this:

### The meeting

We meet at last then. I never thought to
See you, or even to know you, that was for others.
Nothing dramatic or sudden to warn me
Of your presence. You'd been there all along.

Waiting, expecting me not to be so stupid
When you gave me so many hints that you were there.
Now we can be easy with each other.
Let us both be patient for the right time.

Your name is Death, I know, stay if you wish
Be patient with me, and one day we
Might be friends.[8]

In 1998, 24 years after her death, her husband, Ian Roddie, revisited the set of poems she wrote as she was dying and published six, including this, in the *British Medical Journal*. He said, as introduction: "The final poem, 'The Meeting,' was written in hospital after chordotomy to relieve pain caused by spinal metastases some days before she died. It tells of the calm and gentle way she came to terms with her death, and it broke my heart."[7] He also wrote notes to go with the full collection of her poems, intending to publish them to share with his family and children.

The writing of these poems seems to have had a double impact. The therapeutic value to Betty is clear: charting her journey through illness and disability, towards death. The very addressing of Death in this way in writing must have deeply affected her attitude. Ian calls it a "calm and gentle way" to come to terms with death. Leaving her husband these poems was a very important thing for Betty to do. The writing of the supportive and explanatory material by Ian is a work of love and dedication, as well as a lasting and effective memorial.

# Poetry: a different form of communication

## What the poem means

do not say
in words
what a poem means
breathe it
through your body
speak it
with your eyes
touch it
embrace it
walk it
in every step you take
dream it
wake with it
in the moment
here and now

(Margaret Holman)

Writing is more physical than talking, arriving on the page by way of the hand being somehow a less cerebral process than talking. "The poem is a physical process, is bodily exercise . . ."[2] The French poststructuralist feminist writers speak of writing from the body.

> Writing is a primary act. It comes from within. I feel it welling up inside me, growing out of me, transforming itself in language. The still dumb flow of writing passes through my woman's body, searching for words . . . I feel that by writing I continually renew myself and replenish vital forces. I need the incessant movement from body to symbol, from symbol to body; for me the two things are intrinsically linked.[8]

Writing is considerably slower and more effortful than talking, preventing the writer wasting time and effort on peripheral or inappropriate words. It uses words to communicate in a different way from our habitual one and so is less trammelled by the rules and social codes around talk.

Great poems are read again and again because they take us into areas of experience to which we cannot or will never go, or they voice our own experience in the most apt of words. How often do we hear "Oh, I haven't the words to tell you about that – it was beyond words"? Poetry grabs in the guts, forcing concentration on so few words for so long because the writer *has* managed to find some of those words. And this is not only the province of the gifted, great poet: poetry which is useful to the writer, and to an appropriate audience such as a group of hospice patients, can effectively be written without the intense redrafting so often necessary to communicate to a wide audience, as we saw with Muriel. Or reworking can be very useful in the struggle for self-understanding, as it is for Angela Morton.

Poetry writing helped me begin to communicate again after a long period of mental disorder involving many weeks in hospital severely depressed, virtually mute and sometimes paranoid. The journey back towards belonging in the ordinary world seemed unbearably slow, and I believed my delight and ease with language was damaged beyond salvage. When creative writing tutor Graham Hartill suggested making a poem with a repeated word at the beginning of each line, small but persistent bubbles of energy disturbed my lethargy. For days I searched. Three words emerged. I'd found a mantra: *and only when*. I added *I'd lain in severing heat*, then: *and only when I'd lain alone in binding ice / and only when all life and love had lain eclipsed*. I knew this was the voice of biblical Lazarus, returned to life four days beyond death.

By next class I'd written my first poem in almost two years. With the voice of Lazarus, I described a journey through death and entombment to a rebirth; with his acknowledged presence I began to trust my creative imagination again. I witnessed how Lazarus emerged from death through the voices of sisters, disciples, parents, a lover. Confidence grew in my ability to move around, unharmed, within my imagination. I explored Jacob Epstein's making of newly risen Lazarus from stone, and entered into dialogue with him within me. There are now nearly thirty poems: experiences of drawing from them, revision and new writing, are several years on, still alive. (Angela Morton)

Probably the most interesting point about Angela's process for me with the Lazarus poems, was the power released in first acknowledging the metaphor and then *sticking with it*, regarding it as a poetic moment, but then as an archetypal image, which can be explored, *excavated* if you like, and played with, built on, worked on ad infinitum. James Hillman talks about the importance of staying with an image to liberate its meanings, its polymorphous winding sheet. But it's vital always to acknowledge the (at least) dual aspects of this kind of process: an unwrapping, a discovery, yes, but also a making, an invention, a *poiesis*. *Soul making* is an act of surrender, of openness to what the image, the language, itself has to say, and at the same time an act of will, of determination, to get to grips with the work. This creative balancing act is surely in itself an incantation of psychic wholeness. (Graham Hartill)

"Poetry is a distortion of language, the stretching of vocabulary, syntax and rhythm until they form new shapes – the creation of a language within a language",[9] a way of grasping and owning it. Poetry writing has not only effectively been used with patients, but also as a tool in healthcare evaluation.[10] It can also help the clinician.

## Physician-poets: a powerful combination

Through the powers of metaphor, rhythm, rhyme and metre, these (poets) transform the mundane world of doctor and patient. Their words evoke levels of empathy with the predicament of illness to which most of us not endowed with the graces of poetry can rarely ascend. Poetry nourishes the poet's soul and emboldens the poet to break the bonds of ordinary logic and language to fathom a little more of the mystery of human healing. Perhaps, as Hesiod and Pindar opined, the poet's "sweet words" themselves may even heal – if not the patient, then the poet.[11]

This is from the introduction to a volume of poetry by physicians, for whom "both their poetry and their art are inextricably grounded in the realities and urgencies of clinical practice". They have not left medicine for poetry, like Keats did. *The Lancet*'s reviewer, Charles Gropper, commented:

One view of poetry is that all poems are really prayers. The depth of pain that physicians must witness, and that, often, they must partially ignore to function, is evident in these poems... All reveal the intensity of the human experience, whether joyful or tragic, that is the physician's privilege and burden to observe. In these experiences and feelings, these physicians are, in some sense, trying to complete their work of healing.[12]

It has been argued, by three physicians that "the 'something' that is missing (in medicine) is our role as physician healers... the healing effect of the doctor-patient relationship."[13] This, as Hippocrates tells us, can have enormous healing power. Poetry writing can engender greater empathy and understanding of the patient, and of the relationship with the patient. "Medicine and creative writing were inseparable aspects of (poet William Carlos Williams) life. What brought them so closely together was his consistent attempt to express the 'thing' of human relationships, the elusive but deep connection between the self and others, between the self and the world."[14]

The Lancet[15,16] and the Journal of the American Medical Association[17] regularly publish poetry; the British Medical Journal (see above) includes many poems, and I edit a poetry page in every issue of Progress in Palliative Care.[18] The healing art of poetry is becoming a mainstream concern within medicine.

## Candour

At eight years old, his cancer running rampage,
Joe perches on my office sofa edge
Thigh-to-thigh with mom
(who has enjoined with me: "Square with him")

But I beat about the bush a bit,
Then come at last to it: "Joey:
You're going to die, go to heaven."
Words lost in his howl, like a wolf's

The hurling of his body into
The yellow print dress's recesses.
Three minutes at least of this, this keening,
While we eye each other, panicked:

Whatever else was right to do this wasn't it.
Then, as instantly, at a long-drawn-in
Breath's end, he stops, swivels out, flicks a look,
Spots tears on cheeks of mum, dad, nurse, me

Determines he's grieved enough. Time to
Lighten up, knowing me at other times a joker,
A wearer of odd socks, funny noses. He spies
Memos, charts, photocopies, journals –

Jetsam of an urgent life – scattering my carpet,
And becomes the stand-up comic,
Offering his own joke: "Didn't your mom
Tell you to pick up after yourself."[19]

John Graham-Pole, an American paediatric oncologist, discovered poetry helps him in his response to his work.

Many of my poems are requiems, or even celebrations, for individual young people I've known. And they help me look at what has surfaced for me in my relationship with each of them. I have been thinking about why I write poetry and can think of at least five reasons: to reclaim my creative self; to express my feelings; to clarify my thinking; to connect with others; and to develop my philosophy of life.[20]

I have several times given a copy of *Candour* to colleagues despairingly wondering: "How can I teach young clinicians about breaking bad news?". It holds no answers, but does give a graphic example.

Dannie Abse, a Welsh doctor poet, has a large corpus of writing. Here is part of a poem about a brain operation under local anaesthetic, in which his father assisted surgeon Lambert Rogers in 1938, when brain surgery was not well advanced.

If items of horror can make a man laugh
then laugh at this: one hour later, the growth
still undiscovered, ticking in its own wild time;
more brain mashed because of the probe's braille path;
Lambert Rogers desperate, fingering still;

then, suddenly the cracked record in the brain,
a ventriloquist voice that cried, "You sod,
leave my soul alone, leave my soul alone," –
the patient's dummy lips moving to that refrain,
the patient's eyes too wide. And, shocked,
Lambert Rogers drawing out the probe
with nurses, students, sister, petrified.[21]

This four-stanza poem tells the story of this horror-surgery in an unforgettable way; prose would wrap it up in too many words and lose the insistence of rhyme and rhythm.

# Poetic form

"Both poetry and medicine, when properly and honestly practised, are attempts to reintroduce that familiar sense of order into an environment gone out of control."[2] Stravinsky said: "Music has been given to us with the sole purpose of establishing an order in things". Oliver Sacks asserts that one of the therapeutic benefits of music is its narrative nature.[22] My husband will sit down at the piano having been really tense about work. Within seconds he becomes absorbed into the demands of the music, oblivious to everything else; when he stops he is completely refreshed and so am I because I scribble while he is playing. One of my GP writing group members has commented how vital the form of the story is in his writing process: "things come out because the story lets them out". Poetry is a refined form of narrative.

Poetry writing is a staged process: the first expressive and explorative draft is followed by exhaustive redrafting and editing. Redrafting is the disciplined crafting of the poem towards a statement as close as possible to the image in the poet's mind and moulding it towards an appropriate form; editing is sorting out the grammar, punctuation and so on. All these stages can be therapeutic. The first draft can be cathartic; in redrafting the writer refines and clarifies, gaining accuracy of memory or image and self-illumination along with it (the sunset was like a *yawn* – in feeling and look; it was a *red* dress I was wearing that day not *blue*, so I was only five, not seven...); editing is as satisfying as weeding or creating a perfect-looking, smelling and tasting dinner.

Editing and redrafting both involve an awareness of *form*. Poetry can be written in free verse or in strict form – the syllables counted in Japanese haiku, beats counted in metrical verse (iambics, for example), complex rhyme schemes adhered to, set lines repeated in villanelles or triolets. Raphael Campo interrogated himself as to why he writes formal poetry.

> ... all have wondered why I am compelled to write poetry, and especially why I bother with so called formal poetry... It is the surgery I have been performing on myself since I began writing poems, as if I too required assisted breathing the way the patient undergoing an operation to remove a malignant tumour requires the temporary artificial imposition of the innate breathing rhythm... Writing good iambic pentameter feels like putting stitches into the anonymous, eternally gaping wound of being

human, and rhymes can be intertwined like surgical knots...
Rhymes become the mental resting place in the ascending
rhythmic stairway of memory.[23]

Robert Hamberger, another poet to stress the ordering function
of poetry, especially strict forms,[24] wrote a sequence of Petrarchan
sonnets when his friend died of AIDS.[25]

Rhyme and metre are not good places for novice poets to start,
on the whole. Campo and Hamberger are poets experienced in
expressing themselves, as well as in using strict form. Many
beginners think poetry has to rhyme and go *de-dum-de-dum*
(iambics), so they start with strict form as a "must" and then think
of what they can cram into it, thus creating doggerel. Form should
merely increase the impact of the content of a poem. In free verse
beginning poets can listen to their own natural rhythms and get a
feel for what suits them. Reading good contemporary free verse
gives excellent examples.

Many of the patients and clinicians I have worked with, or whose
poetry I have seen, have no knowledge of poetic form yet write first
draft material (sometimes lightly drafted) which communicates,
because they have been willing to pour their experience into it and
accept whatever comes in the way of both content and form.

Life does not come in neat slices like in fiction or poetry. Poetry
cannot be disciplined by the thinking mind of the poet, as one of
my group members, just starting out, realised: "I like poetry
because I can't make it do what *I* want it to do, it will only do what
*it* wants." She added: "I didn't want to write the poem I did write,
I wanted to write a nice glowing poem about being a mother".

I ask people to write whatever arrives at the pencil-point. The
writing may grow up later to become a sonnet or whatever, possibly
with much redrafting. Redrafting can be a vital part of the
therapeutic process: to get as close to the image in the mind as
possible, and to benefit from the sense of order and control offered
by rhyme and metre.

Beginning poets who are keen to write and get published often
think they can imitate the form and bypass the intense experience
required by poetry writing. Poetry is useful as a personally
expressive form because the material for it has to be hauled up as
in a bucket from the deep well of experience.[26] This can require
bravery, because the poet will never know what that bucket will
draw up. There is no bypassing this personally adventurous
approach.

## The slim line between danger and benefit

Here is Lindsay Buckell's account of a group of women health workers who met, with me, over a weekend in a place which was both beautiful and not the working or living space of any of us. These elements all allowed greater scope for depth: our ordinary worlds could recede and we could become immersed in this strange yet safe place with this small group.[27] Written in response to my suggestion of writing from a stranger's point of view, Lindsay chose to write reflexively about us, as if she was a researcher observing our group:

> There is a slope in the green field and a tree standing against the skyline, and over the drystone wall the valley, and more hills beyond. The barn is built of warm limestone, and sitting around a long table are a group of women writing.
>
> They don't know I'm watching them, and that is good, because it's part of the research and, of course, it would make the results all wrong if they knew. I noted in my book last night that they were asked to write about a significant moment when things were different, and this morning to see it from a stranger's view. They don't have to do that if something else seems more important.
>
> I'm stunned really by what I have observed; it looks so hard, this task they have set themselves. They've started, hesitant, not knowing, then I've seen them overwhelmed, sometimes by laughter, often by tears. There have been some memories, thoughts, they've been surprised by how it feels. They didn't know they knew it, thought it, felt it, until it flowed unbidden from the pen.
>
> To me, the researcher, it looks so brave, but what a risk worth taking. I shall have to write in my report about how every moment is significant and how, every moment, life is never the same again. (Lindsay Buckell)

And in a way life never was the same again, particularly for one member of this group.

This kind of writing does change lives. It enables us to listen to what is in our hearts, to still the busy babble of all the everyday things we have to do and think about. A nurse in another group commented: "this is an assertiveness training course". She found herself a better nursing job.

# Poetry for patients

Writing has an evidence base for alleviating the symptoms of anxiety and depression. A report of a randomised control trial has been published,[28] showing how writing about the most stressful event of their lives can create clinically relevant symptom reduction in patients with asthma or rheumatoid arthritis. The opinion in the journal's editorial was: "Were the authors to have provided similar outcome evidence about a new drug, it likely would be in widespread use within a short time."[29] This trial of the therapeutic effectiveness of disclosure writing follows on from a wide range of trials conducted by James Pennebaker et al,[30] all demonstrating significant health benefits to people after writing about their lives" most stressful time.

Healthcare staff can effectively suggest poetry writing to patients.[31] Another excellent book on where to start and how to develop the work is Ann Kelley's Poetry Remedy. She suggests not calling it "poetry": the word can seem scarily difficult or "poetry is for wimps".[6] Also, it is better if beginning poets concentrate on the process of writing rather than worrying about ending up with a product. "It is not the arrival which matters; it is the journeying."[6]

Patients need no special talents or artistic genius but poetry writing is like travelling through a maze. Every turning is a surprise.

Patients need trust in the process of writing, and faith that they can do it. They need to know they must take responsibility for themselves or it will not work. I always explain the presence of a deep, strong, wise, healing voice inside: poetry taps into this. Encouraging them that they won't write the wrong thing can offer confidence and greater self-respect. We are too used to feeling that only proper writers know how to write: that we can't spell, don't know the right forms or clever modes of expression. Whatever is written will be right for each writer and does not have to fit into any canon. The issues, feelings or memories raised by the writing can feel difficult or painful at the time, but I have found that writers feel the struggle to face them is well worth it. If the time is not right for a problematic area to be explored, then, in my experience, they stick to matter-of-fact material or say they don't want to write at all. Anyone who introduces another to poetry writing must try it themselves first, both to gauge their own parameters and boundaries, and to experience the power of self-discovery. I would also advise finding a support person before beginning – someone to talk through what is going on or to take over with the patient if the clinician feels they have gone as far as they can.

Such poetry is generally only written for the satisfaction of the writer and a tiny chosen audience. It does not help if people feel they are competing in the same literary world as Hopkins or Heaney; poetry published for a wide audience takes skill and experience, many hours of hard redrafting, editing, soul and mindsearching and an extensive use of the waste-paper basket. Yet I feel certain poetry, such as Betty Roddie's, written *in extremis*, seems to leap over the necessity for hard work and offer something of intrinsic value. Health professionals can gain from reading the writing of patients, furthermore, gain in companionable and compassionate insight.

## Finally

Learning to live with oneself – in health, sickness and when dying – is not an innately easy process. Private poetry writing and reflection upon that writing can offer insight and guidance, either alone or supported by a practitioner or clinician with experience of facilitating personal development. Poetry can be: cathartically expressive and explorative, a way of testing personal hypothesis, of leaving a record of memories, ideas, hopes, feelings, and of exploring experiences we can never have ourselves, like Betty's poem about death.[7] Writing in this way can offer a sense of control and order, and is enjoyable, exhilarating even. Poetry writing can help one accept life's uncertainty, and face one with oneself. Life's biggest questions will not be answered, The Truth never discovered. But you will find that:

Without going outside, you may know the whole world.
Without looking through the window, you may see the ways of
   heaven.
The further you go the less you know.
Thus the sage knows without travelling.[32]

### Acknowledgements

I would like to thank all the patients and healthcare staff I have worked with, particularly Muriel and Lindsay Buckell (written permission is held for publication of hitherto unpublished material). I would also like to thank Margaret Holman, Ian Roddie,

Kate Billingham, Angela Morton, Graham Hartill, Sam Ahmedzai, Tony Bethell, Nigel Mathers, Marilyn Lidster and Stephen Rowland.

# References and notes

1 *Beowulf* (trans. M Alexander). Harmondsworth: Penguin, 1973.
2 Campo R. *The Desire to Heal*. Norton: New York, 1997: 167.
3 *Hippocratic Writings* (trans. GER Lloyd). London: Penguin, 1950.
4 Maudsley H. In: McDougal J (ed.). *Theatres of the Body*. London: Free Association Books, 1989.
5 Shakespeare W. *Hamlet*: I.iii.75.
6 Kelley A. *Poetry Remedy*. Newmill: Hypatia Trust, 1999: 12.
7 Roddie B. Coming to terms with death. *BMJ* 1999; **317**: 1737.
8 Cixous H. Writing as a second heart. In: Sellers S (ed.). *Delighting the Heart: a notebook by women writers*. London: The Women's Press, 1989.
9 Balmer J. *Sappho: poems and fragments*. Newcastle-upon-Tyne: Bloodaxe Books, 1992: 26.
10 Wilkinson M. *Creative Writing: its role in evaluation*. London: King's Fund Publishing, 1999.
11 Pellegrino ED. Introduction. In: Belli A, Coulehan J (eds). *Blood and Bone: poems by Physicians*. Iowa City: Iowa Press, 1998: xiii.
12 Gropper C. Well versed in medical practice. *Lancet* 1998; **353**: 759.
13 Dixon M, Sweeney KG, Pereira Gray DJ. The physician-healer: ancient magic or modern science? *Br J Gen Pract* 1999; **49**: 309–13.
14 Belli A, Coulehan J (eds). *Blood and Bone: poems by Physicians*. Iowa City: Iowa Press, 1998: xv.
15 Bolton G. A log fire warms you twice. *Lancet* 1997; **349**: 1183.
16 Bolton G. No thank you. *Lancet* 1997; **349**: 217.
17 Smith BH. Old malady. *JAMA* 1995; **274**: 1412.
18 Bolton G. Dregs. *Prog Palliat Care* 1997; **5**: 34.
19 Graham-Pole J. In: Belli A, Coulehan J (eds). *Blood and Bone: poems by Physicians*. Iowa City: Iowa Press, 1998: 27.
20 Graham-Pole J. Children, death and poetry. *J Poetry Therapy* 1996; **9**: 129–41.
21 Abse D. *Collected Poetry*. London: Penguin, 1977: 96.
22 Sacks O. *The Man Who Mistook His Wife For A Hat*. London: Picador, 1985: 176–7.
23 Campo², 102, 116, 166.
24 Hamberger R. Quoted in Bolton G. *The Therapeutic Potential of Creative Writing: writing myself*. London: Jessica Kingsley, 1999.
25 Hamberger R. Acts of parting. *New Statesman* 1995; 24 November: 49; also Hamberger R. *Warpaint Angel*. Leicester: Blackwater Press, 1997: 44–56.
26 Byron C. Writers on teaching. In: Thomas S (ed.). *Creative Writing*. Nottingham: Nottingham University Press, 1995.
27 Bolton G. Every poem breaks a silence that had to be overcome: the therapeutic power of poetry. *Feminist Rev* 1999; **62**: 118–33.
28 Smyth JM, Stone AA, Hurewitz A, Kaeu A. Effects of writing about stressful experiences on symptom reduction in patients with asthma or rheumatoid arthritis. *JAMA* 1999; **281**: 1304–9.
29 Spiegel D. Healing words: emotional expression and disease outcome (Editorial). *JAMA* 1999; **281**: 1328–9.
30 Pennebaker JW, Kiecolt Glaser J, Glaser R. Disclosure of traumas and immune function: health implications for psychotherapy. *J Consult Clin Psychol* 1988; **56**: 239–45.

31  Bolton G. *The Therapeutic Potential Of Creative Writing: writing myself*. London: Jessica Kingsley, 1999
32  Tao Te Ching Feng, GF. *Lao Tsu*. English J (trans). London: Wildwood Haige, 1972.

# 8

# Spirituality as an integral part of healthcare

Ilora G Finlay and Paul Ballard

Healthcare is a misnomer for the services that are encountered by those who are ill. Far from their health status being maintained, investigation and treatment attempt to correct, in part, a disorder that has occurred and which sometimes means that the person's life has been changed irrevocably. For a person with serious illness, it is the very loss of health that imposes emotions of grief as responses to this loss. Both patient and family, and others on whose lives the patient has impinged, experience these feelings. At such times of stress, questions about the meaning of suffering become a natural response by all affected.

Holistic, or whole person, care has been increasingly recognised as important to patient ease because it respects the multifaceted needs of patients as people. Although it has been a term associated with alternative or complementary therapies and with homeopathy, the philosophy is being integrated with the scientific approaches of traditional allopathic western medicine.[1,2] Within the philosophy of holistic care, biopsychosocial needs are reasonably clear and addressed within an interdisciplinary approach.[3] Undergraduates and postgraduates in all disciplines learn about the important physical aspects of providing care and are taught communication skills and about psychological responses to situations. The social needs of patients, including their financial concerns, are recognised as having a profound effect on their ability to be cared for in their own home or in a place of their choosing. Despite the current recognition of the physical, psychological, and social needs of patients, the word "fear" does not feature in the index of standard medical or nursing textbooks. Yet fear is the experience of the majority who enter hospital, even when also tinged with relief at being able to access much-needed help.

Holistic care was developed and pioneered in large part by the hospice movement, founded over 30 years ago when Dame Cicely Saunders started St Christopher's hospice. Since then many Christian religious foundations have established hospices in various parts of the world and a few have secular origins.[4] Pain and symptom control developed as a distinct discipline with recognition that psychosocial distress greatly increases a patient's perceived physical suffering. The underlying physiological mechanisms for these responses have now been explained with, for example, the gate theory of pain.

As physical, emotional, and social needs can be analysed and to some extent quantified, it has become increasingly apparent that a patient's needs in the spiritual domain are less easily defined.[5] The concept of total pain emerged from hospice care, as it became apparent that those who had emotional or spiritual conflicts/concerns exhibited great distress beyond that caused by their physical symptoms. This exacerbation of spiritual distress was evident in those who felt the very essence of their being was threatened by past guilt or conflicting perceptions of impending death and afterlife. However, perhaps as a direct result of the religious base of many hospices, much confusion has arisen between the terms "spirituality", "religion" and "religiousness" in the care of patients.

## Ambiguity in the literature

In general, authors have agreed that the concept of spirituality is broader than religion and there is consensus that religion refers to the doctrine and practice within those formal institutions that we regard as "devotional". Thus, religion focuses on a relationship with God,[6] although our understanding of religion may depend on our understanding of the nature of life.[7] A consensus definition is that spirituality refers to the propensity to make meaning through a sense of relatedness to dimensions that transcend the self.[8]

As we witness others suffering, our own vulnerability is put to the test, raising difficult questions about the meanings and values of different relationships: with self, with others and perhaps with God.[9] In contrast to this personal questioning, theology as a discipline historically has had a bias toward religious systems and beliefs, ignoring these personal and emotional responses to loss.

Frankl[10] has said "Everything can be taken from man but one thing: the last of human freedoms – to choose one's attitude in any given set of circumstances, to choose one's own way". It is this uniqueness of a human's personal choice in thought that perhaps drives many to search for meaning in the midst of suffering. This perception of self is heightened as the sick person becomes aware that his relationship with self is greater than the body, which changes with illness, the mind, which responds to external stimuli or the emotions of a person, as he fluctuates and changes. For it is in witnessing the death of others that we become aware of the terrible finality of death itself and its effects on the bereaved.

The amount of time spent discussing religion and spirituality has, in today's secular society, probably decreased. By contrast, changes in western culture have resulted in open discussion about sexuality, leaving spirituality as the topic that is approached with embarrassment and hesitation or a sense of sceptical disinterest. An increasingly utilitarian approach has promoted the importance of physical perfection with a tendency to stigmatisation of those with physical or psychological disorder. This utilitarian approach has perhaps replaced the concept that, for example, such affliction "is God's will".

However, Walter[11] identified a contemporary approach which balances a religious, ecclesiastical perspective with the perception that the spiritual is the search for meaning.

As society tends to grow more distant from religion as a form of expression of spiritual faith, the spiritual dimension of a patient's perception of self has become increasingly recognised as playing a part in their ability to maintain health. Attention to issues of faith and meaning has also been shown to help those who are ill to cope with disease and respond to treatment.[12] Some striking examples of positive outcomes from the involvement of churches as organisations come from the care of people suffering from various forms of dementia, particularly Alzheimer's disease, who can be helped through one-to-one pastoral visits, which overcome communication difficulties, and by attendance at simple religious services. The move towards biopsychosocial models of care has increasingly recognised the importance of a spiritual dimension to people's lives.[13] Professionals" perceptions and practice of spirituality in caring have been explored in hospices providing care to terminally ill adults,[14, 15] in an oncology setting and in paediatric care.

The nursing, medical, and theological literature on spirituality show a common ambiguity and lack of understanding of the essence of spirituality in care. Spirituality has been dubbed the ignored dimension in healthcare, probably because it cannot be measured and monitored. The medical rationale for this ambiguity in healthcare is that spirituality is not a provable and quantifiable part of care, but is an abstract and less tangible concept. The nursing literature highlights that spirituality is very subjective and personal[16,17] and is influenced by an individual's culture, background, upbringing and social contexts.[18] Several authors[19-23] have emphasised that nurse education pays scant attention to spiritual care and leaves nurses ill prepared to cope with the sensitivity of these needs in their patients.

## Secular society, Christian hospices

Many hospices were founded by those from Christian religious groups, particularly Roman Catholics and Anglicans, and the provision of spiritual care is generally viewed as an integral part of the duties of all hospice professionals.[24,25] This is reflected in a highly motivated workforce and there is evidence that a sense of religious calling or vocation has a positive influence on care giving, which can be harnessed to good effect amongst staff and volunteers. Yet when tested in practice, the behaviour of professionals has been shown to vary according to their discipline, training and role modelling. These influences override experiences of social role, so that nurses and social workers on home visits have been found to address spiritual issues and death anxiety far less than chaplains. However, Hall[26] has highlighted how hospice chaplains, as part of the care-giving team, must understand their own limitations in trying to provide spiritual support to those with differing religious and spiritual beliefs.

Cornette[27] defined the spiritual as that active need within each human being to situate oneself in a horizon that gives meaning to life's experience. This spiritual dimension may use elements such as a holy book or prayer to place the individual in relation to God and to join a group of like-minded people, sharing a moral code. The term "spirituality" has been used synonymously with institutionalised religion,[28,29] as a description of a life force within[30] and as the capacity for transcending in order to love and be loved,[31] but others have stated that spirituality *per se* cannot and should not be equated with religion.[32] Elsdon[33] pointed out that spiritual needs differ from religious needs and inferred that everyone has spiritual needs whether or not they are part of a formal religion.

Until recently, the norms in society tended to restrict the practising of religion to Christianity in its highly institutional forms. Edassey and Kuttierath[34] suggest there is considerable resistance in hospice care to maintaining a non-faith specific outlook, as the concept of spiritual care in hospices still has a predominantly Christian framework, making this spiritual care, as now practised, unsuitable or unacceptable to non-western ethnic groups. Such a restrictive view of care given in a religious framework evidently will fail many patients, even those who have been brought up in the Judeo-Christian framework.

Despite much descriptive work from the professional's perspective, spirituality as a topic has not been researched in great depth from the patient's perspective. This failure to address spirituality as a fundamental component of patient care may have implications for patients' expectations from, and satisfaction with, healthcare delivery within the palliative care setting. As patients experience loss, fear or despair, they may search, sometimes for the first time, for meaning and purpose to their existence, the very existence that is gravely threatened. Therefore a study was undertaken, using focus group methodology, to explore this dimension of personhood from the rich narrative of patients' descriptions of their experiences in a hospice day unit.

## The patients' view

The study aimed to investigate patients' perspectives of pastoral, spiritual and religious needs in a regional palliative care centre (Holme Tower Marie Curie Centre, Penarth, South Wales) and to investigate how patients felt these needs are best met.

A focus group methodology was used as the technique capitalises on the group interaction to elicit rich experiential data, providing insight into beliefs and attitudes that underlie behaviour.[35,36] This method may also be more appropriate in palliative care, as the security of being "in the crowd"[37] provides group support to vulnerable patients.

Patients in day care were approached as they were well enough to participate and were physically able to come to a group. Twenty-nine of the 70 patients attending day care participated in the focus groups of 4–6 participants, held on a series of afternoons at times convenient to the patients. A semi-structured approach, which had been piloted on non-nursing hospice staff, raised consistent areas for discussion within each group. All discussions were tape-recorded, transcribed by an independent medical secretary and analysed for consensus themes, with groups and participants numerically coded.

These patients were all drawn from the postindustrial communities of South Wales, the majority having been resident in the area for many years. From the group emerged a rich history of the Welsh Valleys and the Vale of Glamorgan, with special reference to chapels and churches within the area. There were moving accounts of past bereavements, of the terrible trauma of war and of grinding poverty and hardship. Several participants had been very harshly treated by their church during their childhood, describing, for example, being scolded for not attending mass despite having no shoes to walk there. Several had experienced judgemental attitudes over divorce and had found the church members to be hypocritical, with this harsh moralistic heritage extending to the present day. In contrast, others described attending church as a spiritually uplifting experience which gave them strength to cope with their illness and provided a valuable source of friends.

Almost all patients described past bereavements as powerful influences on their current thinking. Those who had lost a child found their faith in an afterlife was particularly important; the thought that their child was being cared for by God provided comfort from the pain of loss many years after the bereavement.

Half the patients had difficulty defining "spirituality", concurring with the confusion that exists in the literature. Some patients associated the term with paranormal experiences, spiritualism and the occult, such as a "cold wind" or when "the dog follows someone (invisible) across the room"; one patient spoke of Chinese healing.

Humour is a dimension of communication often used to transmit unpleasant as well as pleasant messages. It can be a way of bonding a group and demonstrating camaraderie in the face of a common foe. Interestingly, all groups exhibited much humour, often to relieve tension when a participant had exposed some deeper thoughts or hurt. Each group had its own dynamic, determined by the participants" behaviour and views; one group was very unfocused despite the efforts of the facilitators.

Seafaring analogies were often used to express concepts. This may reflect the setting of the hospice, adjacent to the Bristol Channel along which large ocean-going ships pass at times, a possible nautical background in some patients' families or it may reflect the large number of analogies to fishing that occur in the Bible.

A consistent major theme from all groups was that support from day care was enriching and uniquely met a need. A common bond developed between patients with a sense of affinity, companionship, caring, and humour. Some strong friendships had been forged and several wanted to spend more time together to share experiences and feelings or express emotion without feeling judged.

I think it's just being around people that are in the same boat. We've all got our different problems; it's the same disease, cancer. I think just sitting there; you don't even have to talk to them, just being with them. When I do leave here I do feel a lot more relaxed just being with these people because they seem to relate better... we seem to be an elite [group] compared to everybody else.

And it's the same amongst ourselves. Whoever it is we are all in the same predicament and we have an affinity there.

Other people that have suffered the same as you, it is easy to talk to and you find that you bond with people that have either got cancer, or you know have been diagnosed that they have got cancer, you tend to bond well personally. I tend to bond with somebody that has been diagnosed as having cancer and then try and help through what you have been through and then I find that the two of you have a bond.

All groups cited adverse changes in other interpersonal relationships. Patients described feeling stigmatised by their illness with friends no longer visiting through fear or embarrassment.

It's the people who put pressure on you, not God. So I just have to bundle along in my own way... My best friend, ... she could not cope with it and I haven't spoken to her since two months after I was diagnosed. She just dropped me like that, just couldn't cope with it at all.

Even if they saw me in the street, they'd cross over and go the opposite direction... they were around all of the time, but the minute I was ill I didn't see them... I mean people now when I say I go to Holme Tower on a Wednesday, they all say how long have you got.

People change completely when they know you've got cancer, somebody actually said to me "Oh I do wish you wouldn't say you've got cancer, can't you say you've got something else".

It's a dirty word to some people. I remember when I was going for chemotherapy and people would cross the road and then later on found out it was embarrassment...They are quite disappointed when you are still on your feet 12 months later.

However, a minority had experienced benefits.

I'm enjoying life; make sure that I'm enjoying every bit of it now and have my holidays. There's no pockets in shrouds.

Dominian[38] has described patients as needing faith and hope in a therapeutic relationship with their treating physician. The Oncology Centre was identified as being a "very spiritual place" and one patient had "thanked (the consultant) rather than God" for her response to chemotherapy. A regular thanksgiving service held by staff in the outpatients' area was felt to have enhanced the department, both for those who attended the service and for those not present. This generated a supportive atmosphere where staff were motivated to help and showed empathy with patients.

It's born in them if you like, they are that type of person who's a caring type of person, who wants to care.

However, the majority described sources of hope outside these patient–staff relationships, citing social isolation, feelings of loneliness and lack of hope in their own future as hard to bear.

I think loneliness is the worst thing ever. It's people I need. I need people. The only thing that lacks in my life is company, is friends.

You've got to have hope though haven't you; if you haven't got hope you're lost.

You've got to have something to cling on to.

Patients spoke openly about the rituals around their own death. Some openly discussed having made a will and several had planned or even booked their funeral service.

Hay[31] described spirituality as the capacity for transcending in order to love and be loved. The patients studied described love of the family as the mainstay of spiritual comfort, but this love was not without personal cost to the patient and at times was the source of both comfort and anguish. Many indicated strongly that this love and closeness served as a barrier which hindered them from exploring any issues relating to inner self, feelings, and emotions. All reported a wish to protect the family from upset; some patients strove hard to cover up their own distress and many avoided talking to their spouse for fear of causing upset.

> You find you can't talk to your family about your illness because they can't handle it. It becomes a burden that presses you down sometimes that you just want to scream and shout and tell them how you really feel. But you can't because they just can't cope with it. They are just about hanging on as it is.

> I have always been quite protective about looking after him because I love this man so dearly, I don't want him to be hurt at all, so he doesn't need to know anything.

> My boy said "Why are you always laughing, why are you always smiling?" I said "Because I don't want you to remember me as miserable. I want you to remember me laughing and smiling".

The literature suggests that patients would wish to talk about spiritual issues with staff and that therefore nurses and others should be trained in the topic. However, no patients related having such conversations with staff, but one patient described a deeply meaningful, spiritually important conversation about death with her own son. Another found her husband's physical help had brought them closer together; another found great support and closeness from her brother-in-law who also was diagnosed with cancer.

> We could talk, we knew exactly how each other felt ... sometimes, I mean I would almost have a screaming fit at home, just to myself, not to anybody else, and he would say "I do exactly the same", but he couldn't speak to his wife, because as he said, "they don't really understand exactly how you feel".

Hospital staff were perceived as "too busy to speak to", particularly nursing staff who were seen to be "very busy caring for patients" and "filling out their reports". Not all patients wanted to discuss their concerns, describing it as "inappropriate in our condition" to be asked about fears of dying. The chaplain in day care was valued greatly. He had no barriers to communication; his inability to prescribe or deliver any physical care was a great strength for it meant that his role was clearly defined, so that patients did not feel guilty for taking his time. He was there to listen, to meet their expressed needs. Neither denomination nor sex of the chaplain mattered to the majority; it was the interpersonal skills more than any intellectual learning that was so valued, suggesting that the personality of the chaplain is crucial to delivering an effective service.

Attending day care had been viewed as a turning point in coming to terms with the illness, its confines, and its implications. The religious structure of a short service was valued; many described attending through a sense of obligation, but feeling "better" afterwards. They enjoyed singing old familiar hymns, which provided the sense of connectedness and community identified by Cornette.[27] Although much music has a religious content, many found great spiritual expression in secular music, concurring with the view that music is a potent expression of spiritual memories. For some, calm quietness signalled spiritual peace, particularly when accompanied by someone close, emphasising the power of non-verbal communication.

These patients did not want to talk to "counsellors"; indeed, the term was abhorred. Yet the process of supportive listening, of being able to describe their pasts, to have their experiences recognised as important and of value gave much support to these terminally ill people. The strength of the care they received did not lie solely in the scientific or organisational skills of the staff providing care.

# Conclusion

The very essence of being human was expressed in the rich narrative of the sick person and in the ability of the others to listen. These skills are not measurable in scientific terms. They represent a human judgement of the quality of a relationship and reflect the personal value structure of the individuals concerned. There are no tangible outcomes for those commissioning services, no questionnaires to assess the situation accurately.

As life enters its final phase and the magnitude of the impact of death looms, the human spirit appears more vital than ever. These patients seem to have a heightened awareness all around them. Aspects of the naturally created world, often previously ignored, gained increased meaning and value. Wonderment at the creation of human life inspires respect for the phenomenon of the human spirit.

Yet, beautiful as human life is, it is also frail and vulnerable – therein lies a paradox as we all face our mortality.

# References and notes

1   Berliner HS, Salmon JW. The holistic alternative to scientific medicine: history and analysis. *Int J Health Services* 1980; **10**: 133–47.
2   Noble J. General internal medicine in internal medicine: at the core or on the periphery? *Ann Intern Med* 1992; **116**: 1058-60.
3   National Council for Hospice and Specialist Palliative Care Services. *Specialist Palliative Care: a statement of definitions*. Occasional Paper 8. London: National Council for Hospice and Specialist Palliative Care Services, 1995.
4   St Christopher's information service. *St Christopher's Hospice*. Sydenham, London.
5   Grey A. The spiritual component of palliative care. *Palliat Med* 1994; **8**: 215–21.
6   Mickley J, Soeken J, Belcher A. Spiritual well-being: religiousness and hope among women with breast cancer. *Image: J Nursing Scholarship* 1992; **24**: 267–72.
7   Cook S. Religion. In: Hastings J (ed.). *Encyclopaedia of Religion and Ethics*, vol X. Edinburgh: T and T Clark, 1918.
8   Reed P. An emerging paradigm for the investigation of spirituality in nursing. *Res Nursing Health* 1992; **15**: 349–57.
9   Hilliard N. Spirituality in hospice care. *Palliat Care Today* 1998; **6**: 52–3.
10  Frankl VE. *Man's Search For Meaning*, 5th edn. London: Hodder & Stoughton, 1987.
11  Walter T. Developments in spiritual care of the dying. *Religion* 1996; **26**: 353–63.
12  Hamilton D. Believing in patient's beliefs: physician attunement to the spiritual dimension as a positive factor in patient healing and health. *Am J Hospice Palliat Care* 1998; **15**: 276-9.
13  McKee DD, Chappel JN. Spirituality and medical practice. *J Fam Pract* 1992; **35**: 201–8.
14  Taylor EJ, Amenta M, Highfield M. Spiritual care practices of oncology nurses. *Oncol Nurs Forum* 1995; **22**: 31–9.
15  Dyson J, Cobb M, Forman D. The meaning of spirituality: a literature review. *J Adv Nurs* 1997; **26**: 1183–8.
16  Ross L. The nurse's role in assessing and responding to patients' spiritual needs. *Int J Palliat Nurs* 1997; **3**: 37–45.
17  McSherry W, Draper P. The debates emerging from the literature surrounding the concept of spirituality as applied to nursing. *J Adv Nurs* 1998; **27**: 683-91.
18  Cawley N. An exploration of the concept of spirituality. *Int J Palliat Nurs* 1997; **3**: 31–6.
19  Simpsen B. Nursing the spirit. *Nursing Times* 1998; **84**: 31.
20  Boutall KA, Bozett FW. Nurses" assessment of patients' spirituality: continuing education implications. *Nurse Educ Today* 1993; **13**:196-201.

21  Oldnall A. A critical analysis of nursing: meeting the spiritual needs of patients. *J Adv Nurs* 1996; **23**: 138–44.
22  Piles C. Providing spiritual care. *Nurse Educator* 1990; **15**: 36–41.
23  Narayanasamy A. Nurses" awareness and education preparation in meeting their patients' spiritual needs. *Nurse Educ Today* 1993; **13**: 196–201.
24  Millison M, Dudley JR. Providing spiritual support: a job for all hospice professionals. *Hospice J* 1992; **8**: 49–66.
25  Taylor EJ, Amenta M. Midwifery to the soul while the body dies: spiritual care among hospice nurses. *Am J Hospice Palliat Care* 1994; **11**: 28–35.
26  Hall B. Spirituality in terminal illness: an alternative view of theory. *J Holistic Nurs* 1997; **15**: 82–96.
27  Cornette K. Forever I am weak, I am strong. *Int J Hospice Palliat Nurs* 1997; **3**: 1.
28  Burnard P. Searching for meaning. *Nursing Times* 1988; **84**: 34–6.
29  Labun E. Spiritual care: an element in nursing planning. *J Adv Nurs* 1990; **13**: 314–20.
30  Amenta M. Nurses as primary spiritual care workers. *Hospice J* 1988; **4**: 47–55.
31  Hay M. Principles in building spiritual assessment tools. *Am J Hospice Care* 1989; **8**: 25–31.
32  Ballard P, Finlay I, Searle C, Jones N, Roberts S. Spiritual perspectives among terminally ill patients: a Welsh sample. *Modern Believing* 2000; **41**(2): 30–8.
33  Elsdon R. Spiritual pain in dying people: the nurse's role. *Prof Nurse* 1995; **10**: 641–3.
34  Edassey D, Kuttierath SK. Spirituality in the secular sense. *Eur J Palliat Care* 1998; **5**: 165–7.
35  Asbury JE, cited in Morgan DI (ed.). *Successful Focus Groups – Advancing the State of the Art*. London: Sage Publications, 1993: 412.
36  Carey MA, cited in Morgan DI (ed.). *Successful Focus Groups – Advancing the State of the Art*. London: Sage Publications, 1993: 413.
37  Hansler D, Cooper C, cited in Nyamathia A, Shuler P. Focus group interview: a research technique for informed nursing practice. *J Adv Nurs* 1986; **15**: 128–88.
38  Dominian J. The doctor as a prophet. *BMJ* 1983; **287**: 1925–7.

# Section 3
# Changing Attitudes

*Introduction*                                                      151

9   Portfolio learning: the humanities in medical education    156

10  A pragmatic approach to the inclusion of the creative
    arts in the medical curriculum                              167

11  United in grief: monuments and memories of the
    Great War                                                   177

12  Why medical humanities now?                                 187

13  Medical humanities: means, ends, and evaluation            204

# Section 3
# Changing Attitudes

# Introduction

This third section addresses the way in which exposure to the humanities is being used in undergraduate medical education to affect attitudes, increase interpersonal skills and help medical students develop insight to recognise and cope with emotional responses. These emotional responses occur in themselves, in fellow professionals and in the patients and families they will encounter over their years of practice. Chapters 12 and 13 concern some of the methods and objectives open to humanities subjects in medical education. The section's first three chapters concern some of the emotional challenges for which medical education must aim to prepare the prospective clinical doctor.

Consider today's student entering medical school. This student entering Shakespeare's third age of man usually has little experience of life and death. Yet the early study of anatomy, the first entry into the dissecting room, the history of the person who has died and the pathology witnessed are harsh encounters, similar to an initiation rite, at the start of becoming a "medic". The section's second contributor, Bernard Moxham has, as an anatomist, worked for years on the donated corpses of those who left their bodies to medical science. The mystery and demystification of death which concern him are encapsulated in the project "The Dance of Death", of which Ian Breakwell's "Death's Dance Floor" visual art formed part and which Moxham describes in some detail. The exhibition, simultaneously macabre, amusing and harshly realistic, stimulated viewers to reflect on their own propensity for voyeuristic fascination with and yet revulsion from death. Moxham describes how Breakwell uses the symbolism of the rose window as a Wheel of Fortune to portray the transient fragility of life. A vivid red hue represents blood and flames whilst in the background children chant the familiar rhyme "Ring-A-Rosey", which describes the rash that appeared as a child was struck down by the Black Death. In an age when we have not known hunger first hand, when AIDS was predicted to be an epidemic similar to plague but in the West has been diverted through public education measures and triple therapy, we tend to view sinister rituals that surround death and torture as perverse and distant. But they are on our doorstep; the need for the Human Rights Act is as great now as it ever was. We cannot run away from the uncomfortable feelings that "Death's Dance Floor" invokes.

Most modern TV programmes and films do not confront the

viewer with the awful finality, the irreversibility of death. How many of these young students have grown up watching endless videos in which the heroine or hero (conventionally, the "goodies") escape unscathed from near-death experiences as their opponents (the "villains") die? Grief, if it is portrayed, is confined to black veils at a funeral scene with solemn music. Bernard Moxham's focus is to take these young and naïve students through their first exposure to death and towards the reality of being a doctor.

Prior to this, the section opens with Ilora Finlay's account of how medical students are taken through the course, learning about the impact of disfiguring treatments on people's body image and sexuality, accompanying a cancer patient on their journey of hope and despair that so often ends in death. Finlay describes how the integration of the experience of others, described in literature, poetry, film, art, and music, allows the student to contextualise, understand, and cope with the raw emotions they may witness at first hand. Newer free-form student-directed learning is collated into a portfolio of experiences, linked to the biomedical knowledge that is essential for accurate diagnostic synthesis, to prepare the newly graduated doctor to make ethically grounded management plans in dialogue with their patients. For Finlay, the change from factually overloaded curricula to recognising the richness of human experience expressed outside the biomedical textbooks gives hope that the next generation of doctors will have those human qualities of empathy and understanding so needed by vulnerable patients. The communication skills required of entrants to medicine, that are taught through the course and the stringent principles of the General Medical Council, are changing the type of graduate for the better. These more sensitive graduates will be more vulnerable emotionally, they will need more support, need to be recognised as humans and they are more vulnerable to the slings and arrows of the media and the lawyers than before.

In the UK today very few of us have had to live through war. We have not experienced the daily reporting of our young and strong, in the prime of life, being cut down by mine, shrapnel or disease. We have not waved our sons off, never to return, to a time of despair and desperation in the cold mud of futile First World War battlefields. We have not sent them to save our land and our people from Nazism. Yet on our doorstep other tragedies have decimated our communities: Aberfan's children killed in a mudslide of coal slag, Lockerbie's air disaster, the IRA bombs...Today little bunches of flowers at the roadside mark a child, a senseless victim of a drunk or distracted driver. Angela Gaffney examines how a community copes with grief, how memorials are central to the grieving process, in her exploration of the way in which that most poignant of emotions, the grief of a parent for their child, has been harnessed, valued, and respected by those communities decimated by the loss of their sons in war. Lack of a well-designed, visually appropriate memorial implies lack of respect to those cut down in their prime. She looks at their importance for a community to function after a disaster, for the grieving to be able to focus their despair and find meaning and hope in their loss. These same memorials serve as permanent reminders of our mortality, our debt to others. They confront us with the value of our freedom and our life – "Lest we forget" is surely apt. All these phenomena are of inescapable importance to the practising doctor, above all the doctor working in a community context. Understanding them involves understanding and appreciating the links between morbidity, mortality, social context and the influence, upon the patient's self-perceptions, of their perspectives, attitudes, and beliefs, in which the community context may play a hugely significant part. There is a need for these matters to be confronted and dealt with seriously in medical education and Gaffney's discussion offers an example of the kind of examination of community issues and perceptions with which the medical student – and indeed the qualified practitioner – could valuably engage.

What is the specific contribution of the humanities to the way in which medical education responds to these challenges? This section's fourth and fifth chapters concern this question directly.

Jane Macnaughton begins by examining the recent rise of medical humanities, asking why they are important now and how they stand in relation to the parallel development of an interest in arts and health. She identifies "arts and health" as having three expressions: in arts therapies proper, in the *ad hoc* involvement of arts in existing therapies, and in the use of arts in community development. The last of these responds to the recognition of social exclusion as a determinant of ill health. The "arts and health", movement thus seems highly distinct from the medical humanities whose initial focus is perhaps on medical education. Even so, they have common roots in responses to the recognition of the socioeconomic factors in health and illness, requiring both a broader range of therapeutic and preventive strategies and a broader based medical education, enabling doctors to work in new and different ways.

Specifically, doctors need to be able to extend beyond biomedicine in their understanding and to apply the technologies of biomedicine in a more humane way. To achieve this, Macnaughton argues that humanities subjects provide sources of case material and demonstrate the nuances of interpersonal communication (*pace* Downie – see below – she holds that they contribute to a development in the *person* who, through encountering them, is educated as well as simply trained). Moreover, they provide the experience of a "counterculture" to medicine, reducing the traditional isolation of medical students from the students of other disciplines.

Macnaughton concludes by distinguishing a third conception of the medical humanities, in addition to the "additive" and "integrative" conceptions which this volume proposes and which Greaves explores in his opening chapter. A "complementary" conception involves juxtaposing the conventional medical viewpoint with other viewpoints, for the student's consideration – "holding up a mirror to the medical view of the world". This model (argues Macnaughton), whilst less radical than the integrative, actually better describes the bulk of medical humanities teaching as it is currently conducted – though whether further evolution is desirable is left an open question.

Finally, then, what are the aims of the humanities in medical education and how is their fulfilment to be gauged? Robin Downie's examination of these questions starts with a wry question which, one may conjecture, stems from experience: how is a sceptical Dean of Medicine to be convinced of the value of medical humanities teaching? The variety of humanities disciplines vitiates their having common aims or evaluations and to be versed in the humanities is demonstrably not the same as being humane.

Downie distinguishes a number of aims for the medical humanities, including the fostering of "transferable skills" such as those of analysis and sensitivity to nuances of argument or varieties of evidence; a "humanistic perspective" including moral sensitivity; the ability to deal with complex situations beyond the reach of protocols or guidelines, drawing upon an understanding of qualitative distinctions; and awareness of self and of one's own emotions. Evaluating these may draw on the traditional humanities methods of tasks in discursive writing, but these must be assessed in a way that is sensitive to the more slender background and immersion in such subjects at the disposal of the typical medical student. Moreover, not all the "skills" transfer equally readily to the medical context and whilst the capacity for a particular humanities study to "make a better professional doctor" is a reasonable focus for a medical Dean, work has to be done to compensate for the variation in how these skills arise out of the associated study of humanities. Downie turns this to advantage in stressing the importance of ambiguity in both the humanities and "the words of patients".

He proceeds to argue that we should decline the familiar distinction between the intrinsic and instrumental values of humanities study, pointing out that humanities study, worthwhile for its own sake, plays a constitutive or "component" role (rather than a merely instrumental one) in the development of the educated doctor. As Downie points out, we too often neglect the question of whether a good doctor needs also to be an educated human being yet "considered judgement" is one hallmark of both.

Collectively, the chapters as a whole reflect medical education's contemporary search for the constituents of "considered judgement"; the present section is concerned with the ground upon which that judgement will need to stand, including the sensitivity and emotional maturity which must be nurtured in today's medical students.

# 9

# Portolio learning: the humanities in medical education

Ilora G Finlay

The humanities have, during the modern era of scientific medicine, been substantially excluded from medical education. Medicine has been deemed the art of the sciences and the science of the arts. Despite the increasing pressure for evidence-based medicine, there is remarkably little understanding of the causes of the majority of "illnesses" and little understanding of how environment, stress, and emotion alter people's responses to their "ill health".

Within the humanities there are rich descriptions of suffering and expressions of emotion in response to life events, both good and bad. Anecdotally we talk of "time as a great healer", "a trouble shared is a trouble halved" and are all aware of those people who "enjoy ill health", with so much gain from being in the sick role that they cannot afford to be well. Sometimes the threat of losing benefits, mobility allowances, etc. can hinder a rehabilitation programme of a person who has been ill for some time. It can be terrifying for someone who has lost confidence to face having to look for work, losing money as benefits are cut and hence drop their standard of living, which is already very low.

So how can medical and nursing students learn about the complexities of the human condition? A biomedical education cannot equip young people in their late teens or early 20s to understand the reactions of a bereaved person, the reactions of someone terrified to learn they have a life-threatening condition or the devastation of long-term disability.

The General Medical Council published a document, *Tomorrow's Doctors*,[1] which has had substantial implications for all medical school curricula. It called for a decrease in factual overload, increased communication skills training and tuition in ethics. The result has been an integration of clinical with the early basic sciences teaching. And excerpts of outputs from the humanities are increasingly seen as useful teaching tools. Their language provides rich metaphorical or symbolic representation, from the patient's and family's perspective, of reactions to disease and loss. New projects have developed. These teach students through the medium of the humanities, such as the new "Literature and Medicine" special study module, integrate humanities through portfolio learning and illustrate the biomedical model with extracts from the humanities.

For example, the film *Cat on a Hot Tin Roof* portrays alcoholism more eloquently than any textbook. Denis Potter's description of psoriasis in the television series *The Singing Detective* allows the viewer to understand the devastating effect of widespread skin disease. A self-portrait by Leonardo da Vinci showing a small basal cell carcinoma on the right cheek beneath the right eye is better drawn and more memorable than a textbook illustration.

The word "fear" does not appear in the index of any of the major medical or psychiatry textbooks. Yet anyone who has been seriously ill will describe fear at some time and the way it affected his or her ability to cope with what was happening. Dannie Abse's poetry is a powerful and spine-chilling expression of the fear of neurosurgery and of other hospital procedures. The book and film *Angela's Ashes* are powerful descriptors of grinding poverty and social inequity. *To Kill A Mocking Bird* gives insight into rape, racial prejudice, and the sociological reaction to psychiatric disease. On a lighter note, in *Winnie the Pooh*, Eeyore is surely a depressive and Tigger could be described as manic. Sylvia Plath's *The Bell Jar* describes depression and her anhedonia preceding her own suicide, whilst in the painstakingly written book *The Diving-Bell and The Butterfly* (*Le Scaphandre et Le Papillon*) Jean Dominique Bauby vividly describes the effect of being completely locked in through neurological damage, as he is only able to communicate through an eye movement. Kafka's *Metamorphosis* tackles stigma and the difficulties of change. *Fly On, My Sweet Angel* by Betsy Anderson gives insight into the devastation of a child's death; surely no-one should be telling a parent of any age of this ultimate tragedy – the death of their child – without some understanding of the import of their words and the phenomenal devastation of the grief and loss. In *Jane Eyre*, Jane's friend dies of tuberculosis. Both Candide's tutor and Pandarus in *Troilus and Cressida* contract syphilis, which is described in the texts. *The English Patient* by Michael Ondaatje describes total dependence on a nurse following severe burns. Dylan Thomas describes vividly the internal emotional conflicts in facing death, a situation we must all encounter but we usually conduct our lives in denial of this reality. The neurologist Oliver Sacks has written books about neurological disorders including Tourette's and other syndromes, described in *The Man Who Mistook His Wife for a Hat*. His book *Awakenings*, also made into a popular film, vividly describes the response of postencephalitic Parkinsonism to the drug L-dopa. Other important modern classics include *Last Orders* by Graham Swift, which is funny and touchingly profound as it explores how we live and how we die. *The Magic Mountain* by Thomas Mann relates the dangers of moral decay and the opportunities for self-discovery during lengthy stays in a Swiss tuberculosis sanatorium and *Cancer Ward* by Solzhenitsyn links the experiences and the despair of the terminally ill in Russia with the despair arising from police control of the state.

In the visual arts, powerful images portray "medical" conditions. Frida Kahlo, a 20th-century artist, repeatedly paints pictures of her feet. Those feet were damaged by polio in childhood and then a bus accident fractured her skeleton and left her in unremitting pain; more than 30 operations followed, but to no avail. To convey unhappy feelings, she painted herself weeping. To project her physical suffering, she showed herself bleeding or with a pole slammed through her body, almost forcing the viewer to experience her own pain and contemplate its impact.

Amongst recent films, *Philadelphia* describes a young man dying from AIDS and in *Erin Brockovich* the community poisoned by radioactive waste in the water go on to contract cancers, giving the viewer a detailed insight into the effect of developing malignancy. *Love Story* portrayed a young woman dying of leukaemia; the more recent film *Rain Man* depicts autism. Mahler's sixth symphony represents death and dying through music. Shostakovich's Leningrad symphony evokes the physical terror felt as an invading army approaches, bringing wounding, death and pain; it has great relevance to refugee and battle medicine today.[2] And so the list of teaching material for medicine goes on and on.

## Portfolio learning

Portfolio learning was initially pioneered by GPs who were tired of conventional postgraduate education programmes, which seemed to have little relevance to their daily work and certainly lacked any interaction or creativity. At the University of Wales College of Medicine the principle of portfolio learning was adopted and developed as part of the postgraduate distance learning course for the Diploma in Palliative Medicine, which started in 1989. Since then it has been used to underpin two major undergraduate projects in the undergraduate medical school: the oncology project in the third year and the final year medicine in the community placement.

The concept of a personal learning portfolio embraces two major dimensions, both of which are narrative undertakings:

- the educational evolution of the author
- a chronological series of commentaries on patients and their families undergoing care.

Students describe their learning with illustrations from any source, which can reveal the depth of the personal education process. Recently read reference material from medical texts often exerts a less powerful influence on the student than television documentaries or newspaper articles. Films, books, poetry, music, artworks, and other visual stimuli may all be potent sources of learning and directly relevant to the problems of the patient being studied.

Sequential contacts with families provide an obvious living source of material for study, as are cases seen in a clinic or on home visits. Those patients who have lived through major historical events in their lives, such as the troubles in Northern Ireland or the last world war, will have their stories to tell. But so do others, for each person has had a unique set of life experiences which are the rich backdrop to their personality and explain their reactions and their beliefs. The student collects and explores them in their historical or social context and links them to the patient as a person. The final product in the narration of the portfolio reveals an evolution of thought and expression, as well as knowledge and skill, and can become a reference source of permanent value to the student as it is so personalised.

There are no rules as this is a learner-centred opportunity for self-expression and creativity, except that patient confidentiality must be meticulously observed and plagiarism is not allowable in any form. The student is encouraged to keep sequential rough notes on the patient's progress, their contacts with the patient and on thoughts and reflections as they observe the patient. There are clinical milestones that act as triggers for learning. Sometimes students record in diary form their thoughts after a difficult conversation or write about how they "wind down" or "de-stress" at the end of the day. Some adopt a "box file" approach, collecting anything that seems relevant and later sorting it into order as the case is written up with its accompanying critique.

In compiling a portfolio the student describes the clinical scenario, paying attention to the biological, psychological, social, and spiritual aspects of the case. The student is required to reflect on what has been observed, describing what was done well, what could have been done differently and to provide evidence for this from any source. The student is expected to demonstrate an understanding of the difference between doctor-centred and patient-centred approaches. For any communication skills to be developed, the student must be able to express thoughts and feelings coherently, clearly and in a way that is acceptable to whoever he or she is addressing. Again, the language of literature has much to inform the process of developing insight into effective communication skills.

The ethical issues of the case study are emphasised throughout the project, including the importance of human values and the individuality of the value placed by a patient on one or another aspect of their life. These concepts of value, and of the non-tangible benefits to be gained from an aspect of care, are drawn from the humanities and are in large part absent from medical texts.

## Year 3: oncology

In most medical schools until recently, oncology and palliative care were not itemised as specific topics; they were supposed to be taught within the different subjects such as medicine, surgery, gynaecology, etc. However, they were poorly taught and focused on the biology of cancer, often missing out psycho-oncology and palliative care completely. Yet one in four of the population will die from cancer and one in three will have a malignancy diagnosed at some time in their lives.

In the third year of study at the University of Wales College of Medicine, the oncology project runs in parallel with other parts of the curriculum over six months.[3] Students are allocated in small groups of 6–8 to a personal tutor whose role is as a facilitator and support in learning; these tutors are drawn from a wide range of disciplines, from oncology and palliative care to general practice and dermatology. The student is allocated a patient and is expected to get to know the patient in the context of their family, to accompany the patient to hospital, to the GP or when investigations are done, in the process learning about the patient's experience of the care system. Waiting in outpatients for the results of a scan or blood test has given students insight into the fear and stress associated with what would otherwise seem a routine outpatients attendance. All this is linked to reading about the biology of cancer itself, so the increase in factual knowledge is mirrored by a developing insight into the patient's perception of the disease and its treatment. The student is expected to follow the patient through the course of six months of the illness, being given credit for the effort they go to in trying to keep track on events and visit the patient. If the patient dies, the tutor's role is to encourage the student to attend the funeral if appropriate, to contact the family in bereavement and to show respect for the person who has died. Patients, when given bad news, have often been amazingly open with the student allocated to them and this has resulted in the student developing a great deal of insight. The importance of hope and of truth telling is often brought home sharply.

## Final year: medicine in the community

In the final year students are on placement throughout Wales; they are expected to fill gaps in their previous education and to ensure a firm grounding in the disciplines of general practice, psychiatry, community paediatrics, and palliative care. The outline format is "The Seven Ages of Man" with a template of areas to be covered in each "age". At the end of the three months of placements, the students come together and are expected to create a teaching session on the salient features of one "Age of Man". Over the course of two days they work in groups of 10–12 to produce a half-hour presentation.

Throughout the placement the students are asked to keep a log of four cases. These are written up in depth and put in the context of the patient, their family and society as well as covering the biomedical and therapeutic aspects of the condition. Students are expected to integrate many different sources of learning into the project. Although the majority of students use only the written word, some have produced powerfully drawn or photographic illustrations of their experiences.

Recent examples of the creativity displayed include a Christmas time presentation of the process of antenatal screening for risk factors in pregnancy and associated investigations, presented as "Mary visiting the antenatal clinic". Another well-scripted play illustrated the importance of skills in breaking bad news and gave the salient features of pointers to a more empathic approach. The problems of cardiovascular disease in mid-life were presented as a "chat-show" with one student being the expert opinion and giving detailed facts about different aspects of heart disease, whilst the role-played characters exhibited resistance to changing their disease-prone lifestyles. Reactions to grief and loss were depicted as a psychotherapy session in heaven; diverse players included a young person killed in a road accident, an elderly lonely lady who died alone in a nursing home, a young woman who died leaving small children behind and a musician post-suicide, whose life had been destroyed some years previously by losing an arm in an accident.

## Year 2: sexuality

A difficult and sensitive subject to teach is that of sexuality and the effect of radical treatments on a patient's perception of self. Students are only just coming to terms with their own sexuality, body image, and sexual feelings; indeed, some in the class may be quite sexually inexperienced and feel very embarrassed at the topic. Yet students need to be prepared for their role as doctors, when they will have to be able to warn patients preoperatively about possible sexual dysfunction after pelvic surgery, about hair loss following chemotherapy for cancer and discuss such mutilating surgery as mastectomy or head and neck surgery.

Experiential learning has much to offer. Students handle breast prostheses, try on skullcaps to see how they would look with no hair, handle stoma bags of different types and learn about the incidence and type of sexual dysfunction following different treatments. They reflect on their own feelings about disability and body image and are encouraged to discuss openly ways of helping patients express their fears.

## Literature and Medicine: a special study module

An optional special study module on Literature/Culture and the Practice of Medicine has recently been introduced for third year students. The course module aims to enhance an understanding of illness and the disease experience through literature and other cultural means. This is achieved through the following subsidiary aims:

- attempt to understand different lay perceptions of illness/disease
- to explore the integration of illness/disease into a social context
- to examine representation of the role of the doctor in literature and more general culture
- to understand ethical issues as discussed in general culture and related to human rights
- to examine representations of metaphor of illness as a potent social comment.

The nine-week block is split into three segments. The first three weeks focus on seminars on mental health, cancer, death and dying, ethics, addiction, doctors and magic, what good is a bad doctor, patients' perception of chronic illness, medicine as an instrument of the state and the book *Doctor Jekyll and Mister Hyde*. The seminar on doctors in literature includes a visit to a coal mine, as AJ Cronin's book *The Citadel* is studied. After this initial intensive period of seminars, most work is at an individual level, with supervision from a tutor. At the end of the middle three-week period the student leads a seminar on their topic of study; formative assessment and full feedback help the student towards their written report. At the end of the module the students" 4000-word essays on their chosen subjects are independently marked.

## Teaching communication skills

Role play is used by many medical schools now to teach communication skills, particularly how to break bad news, to obtain informed consent and to cope with an angry or depressed patient or relative. Role play is powerful and requires careful supervision and firm boundaries, or rules, to ensure that no participant feels emotionally damaged or exposed by the experience.

Many students enter medical school with preconceived ideas of how they should behave as a doctor, based on their own personal encounters with medical care or on a perhaps fictional role portrayed on television or other drama, which may need to be modified. It is worth considering, though, that patients themselves often play roles they perceive they should have, often "learnt" from television and informed by what is authentic to their own experience.

"Sculpting", a theatrical technique, has been used in postgraduate education to highlight ethical dilemmas. A group of trained actors play out a scene drawn from real cases and the audience of students is invited to comment on the thoughts, the actions, and the processes portrayed. They can even, as a group, suggest responses, the next line or different actions and then can see the scene unfold. It is a powerful teaching tool, particularly when a large group covers communication skills, ethics or complex psychosocial aspects of care. It allows the participants to share experiences and expertise, to learn from each other and can be very cost efficient as a teaching method. The power of theatre, which communicates with many simultaneously, is harnessed to influence the individual by actively involving them in a situation of direct personal relevance.

# Does all this produce a different type of doctor?

All this is far removed from the rigid sciences of biochemistry, anatomy, and physiology of past years, from the taboos and suppression of emotion associated with the medical curriculum and the bravado of students renowned for drinking too much and playing rugby. Yet how can these changes be evaluated, as there is no randomised controlled trial of undergraduate medical education being undertaken and the changing demands of society are forcing a rapid pace of change? There is some, but not conclusive, evidence that the students educated in the new problem-orientated or integrated curricula may have better diagnostic skills than those from a conventional style curriculum,[4] and in their first clinical year they appear to have improved communication skills.[5]

The General Medical Council will now demand revalidation.[6] The number of complaints against doctors has risen and some have been very public. Assessment of communication skills and evidence of a grounding in reflective practice support the premise that today's medical graduate has received a very different type of education. The challenge is to ensure diagnostic and technical skills are preserved and improved within this holistic approach. Only then can standards improve.

The type of student offered a place at medical school is also changing, bringing a wider background experience to the cohort of students. Excellence in the humanities is welcomed at A level, particularly English, History, Religious studies or another language, with an "arts" subject carrying equal weight to a science subject. The University of Wales College of Medicine has deliberately widened access as the new half and full advanced level courses are introduced, to include the humanities subjects and general NVQs as eligible entry criteria.[7]

And locally in Wales the evidence of a different type of graduate is emerging. It is only anecdotal at present, but tutors of final-year students have remarked on their ability to show compassion and to communicate effectively, their understanding of the gravity of medical decisions and their insight into human suffering. The students" own evaluations of their placements also indicate the powerful learning experience, for many, of this exposure, particularly in primary care.

There are major implications for those involved in the selection of applicants for medical school. Do those with a broad educational base as school leavers carry a breadth of vision through into their clinical practice? Are their learning styles intrinsically different[8] from those of the medical school entrants of yesteryear? Perhaps these questions must be answered with a degree of urgency. The danger is that the graduate may not fit the high-tech demands of molecular science; this just might replace the problems associated with the poor communicators of the past. The challenge is therefore to achieve the right balance to ensure that medicine as a discipline enhances the physical, psychological, and social health of the nation.

# References and notes

1   General Medical Council. *Tomorrow's Doctors: recommendations on undergraduate medical education*. London: General Medical Council, 1993.
2   The Royal Society of Medicine now has a section on "Catastrophe and Conflict" to bring together all healthcare-related disciplines interested in providing relief medical services.
3   Finlay IG, Maughan TS, Webster DJT. Portfolio learning: a proposal for undergraduate cancer teaching. *Med Educ* 1994; **28**: 79–82; Finlay IG, Maughan TS, Webster DJT. A randomised controlled study of portfolio learning in undergraduate cancer education. *Med Educ* 1998; **32**: 172–6.

4   Schmidt HG, Machiels-Bongaerts M, Hermans H, ten Cate TJ, Venekamp R, Boshuizen HPA. The development of diagnostic competence: comparison of a problem-based, an integrated, and a conventional medical curriculum. *Acad Med* 1996; **71**: 658.

5   Rolfe IE, Andren JM, Pearson S, Hensley MJ, Gordon JJ. Clinical competence of interns. *Med Educ* 1995; **29**: 225–30.

6   General Medical Council. *Proposals for Revalidation.* London: General Medical Council, 2000.

7   University of Wales College of Medicine. Prospectus for A104 and A106 courses, 2000–2001.

8   Kolb D, Rubin IM, McIntyre JM. *Organisational Behavior: an Experiential Approach.* Englewood Cliffs: Prentice-Hall, 1994.

# 10

# A pragmatic approach to the inclusion of the creative arts in the medical curriculum

Bernard Moxham

> The medical establishment has become a major threat to health.
> The disabling impact of professional control over medicine has
> reached the proportions of an epidemic.[1]

Many within the medical profession feel themselves to be increasingly maligned. They believe that the profession's reputation has changed considerably in recent times and certainly very markedly from the time when Voltaire wrote "Men that are occupied in the restoration of health to other men by joint exertion of skill and humanity are above all the great of the earth". The reasons for the change in reputation are undoubtedly many and various. At a period when patients are very knowledgeable about medical matters, and when they are more and more willing to assert their rights of "ownership" of their bodies, doctors cannot expect their medical opinions to go unquestioned.

Furthermore, the very success of therapeutic and preventive medicine in controlling (and sometimes eradicating) so many infectious diseases, providing effective contraceptive measures, improving obstetric care and providing fertility counselling and treatment, diminishing neonatal and infant mortality, improving surgical treatments, and understanding and treating the aged and terminally ill has engendered unreasonable expectations for "perfection" in healthcare, for improved longevity and active life in old age, and for the rapid development of treatments for newly emerging, major diseases (e.g. AIDS). Also, perhaps unreasonably, with the decline in religion and the search for sympathetic persons to provide pastoral care, doctors are increasingly being required to act as counsellors. Thus, the demands nowadays placed upon medical practitioners to be good scientists, infallible diagnosticians, successful treaters of disease, counsellors and "opinion makers" are perhaps beyond normal human endeavour. In addition, social critiques (such as those provided by Illich),[1] too often eagerly seized upon by some politicians and bureaucrats, aim not just to bring about a democratisation of medicine and to understand its limits but also, indirectly, to diminish the importance of the profession and of its political "power base".

Antiscientific attitudes have further contributed to the change in the medical profession's reputation and these attitudes have become more vociferous and belligerent as medical science has become more and more successful. Cultural theorists have also added to the demeaning of scientific medicine by referring to it merely as one more "social construct" of no greater significance than any other such "construct"! As asked provocatively by the author Robertson Davies: "How can a doctor possibly be a 'humanist' in a society that increasingly tempts him (sic) to be a scientist?".

Given these circumstances, it is perhaps not surprising that the medical profession sometimes adopts an overly defensive position and appears, on occasion, to dismiss contemptuously those who criticise it. And yet, in my experience, members of the medical profession contribute some of the most humane, intellectual and cultured members to our society. Indeed, it is appropriate to record here that, amongst the students that I have taught, there have been many international sportsmen and women, numerous musicians (including a Yale harp and organ scholar), and many writers, poets, and visual artists.

Even a brief trawl through a list of distinguished writers brings up many who had medical training, including Oliver Goldsmith, Tobias Smollett, Keats, Dannie Abse, William Carlos Williams, Breton, Aragon, and James Joyce. Furthermore, there are many existing examples of the incorporation of the arts into the medical curriculum. This chapter provides just one example of how, within Anatomy at Cardiff University, medical scientists and creative artists have collaborated to deal with the issues surrounding human mortality. My purpose essentially is to show that such collaborations, based primarily upon creative rather than critical operations, can advance the standing of medicine.

# The Dance of Death

With the artist Ian Breakwell, Cardiff has received a Wellcome Trust grant (under its SCI-ART scheme) to develop our project on the theme of mortality. This project we have termed "The Dance of Death" and it has several elements. First, we have produced over 20 works of art which utilise modern medical imaging technologies and these have featured in a touring exhibition ("Death's Dance Floor") with an accompanying, fully illustrated catalogue. Second, we are assessing (via questionnaires) attitudes towards death amongst medical students, the chronically and terminally ill, and amongst the population in general. Third, the material from the project will be transferred to CD-ROM. Amongst its uses, the CD-ROM will create an opportunity for members of the lay population and the medical profession alike to have a suitable vehicle for discussion of the theme of mortality.

Underlying our project is the belief that contemporary western culture, based largely upon secular and materialistic visions, has effectively denied the possibility of intelligent and informed discussion of mortality and has relegated the topic to a status less than that of a taboo. Indeed, it seems that a fixation on the unbridled and inherently selfish pursuit of happiness, together with the hegemony of the "cult of youth", has led to our being consigned to live in an age of *carpe diem* ("seize the day"). As a consequence, death is considered to have been "tamed" and we are left with a culture that is so excessively life affirming that notions relating to death only attract resentment. This is perhaps ironic, given the fact that mass tragedy appears to be our daily diet on television and in the newspapers. Death is everywhere but nowhere!

In his influential essay on death ("The pornography of death"), Geoffrey Gorer[2] argues that, whilst consciousness of death was very much part of life in most cultures, death in the "developed" world has become an "obscene" subject. Thus, we have come very far from Schopenhauer's belief that, after overcoming the powerful but irrational urge to live, we welcome the release of death. More recently, Phillipe Ariès[3] claims that death has been "banished" so that people in urban environments proceed with their daily lives as if nobody died any more. For most of today's urban dwellers (and increasingly for many in the rural population), death therefore appears to be unrepresented and unrepresentable in contemporary culture. That the graveyard is no longer culturally and geographically centrally placed but is peripheral and kept well out of sight, is a sign of our lack of regard for, and confidence in, issues relating to mortality. Even within the confines of the family, where once the death of a relative required the observance of generally approved religious, cultural and social rites (including the laying out of the body within the family home), death is denied and is a despised visitor. In our time, death tends to occur in places remote from the individual's real home (in hospitals, hospices, nursing homes), the undertakers "deal" with the unpleasantries, the body need not be seen, and the deceased is buried or cremated with the minimum of fuss. Dying has become an alienating experience that we wish to ignore. According to Walter Benjamin, "Dying was once a public process in the life of the individual and a most exemplary one; think of the medieval pictures in which the deathbed has turned into a throne toward which the people press... In the course of modern times, dying has been pushed further and further out of the perceptual world of the living. There used to be no house, hardly a room, in which someone had not once died... Today, people live in rooms that have never been touched by death, dry dwellers of eternity."[4]

It is perhaps particularly within the medical profession(s) that mature reflection on the issues is most needed. Today's medical education seems to instil in doctors the notion that death is the enemy and doctors too frequently regard the death of their patients as professional failure. Indeed, to quote Illich once more, "Through the medicalization of death, healthcare has become a monolithic world religion" where "technical death (defined by the medic) has won its victory over dying".[1] These notions become particularly acute with the loss of dissection room teaching of anatomy in the medical curriculum and the fashion of trying to teach the subject by hi-tech means. Furthermore, while it is relatively easy to teach doctors how to inform patients and their relatives about terminal illness, without the doctor understanding mortality (and particularly their own), the maturity needed to empathise with the patients will be missing. A mature understanding of death would be welcome for all. How should such maturity be measured? Both individually and collectively, by the degree to which death as an inevitable outcome for all beings and for all things is accepted; life should be understood as much in terms of death as in terms of life. This of course is not a comfortable concept. Yet, in an age of *carpe diem*, how is it possible for the individual to be other than selfish and how is it possible for a society to progress?

Artworks concerned with the theme of death were predominant during the Middle Ages and the Renaissance. However, many notable attempts to deal with the theme in the visual arts during the 20th century have primarily related to the realities of war and the irrational concerns of the surrealists. For contemporary artists, the attraction of dealing with death is often the attraction of dealing with a taboo. In its western usage, "taboo" has become a non-statutory inhibition on the use of specific words and images, based upon the notion of common decency which, if broken, provokes moral outrage. Little wonder, therefore, that artists wishing to question matters relating to morality, notions of common decency and bourgeois values have found taboos associated with death fertile ground for their work. The dilemma, of course, is that such confrontation can reinforce moral outrage and thus discourage meaningful discussion of issues. Alternatively, the work might appeal only to admirers of the grotesque and thus encourage voyeurism and/or prurience. A selection of contemporary art concerned with death can be found in a variety of exhibitions and books. These include "Vile Bodies"[5] on Channel 4 television, "Don't Leave Me This Way" curated by Ted Gott,[6] and in Deanna Petherbridge's survey of artists and anatomy "The Quick and the Dead".[7] Such ideas, whilst inviting a new aesthetic and questioning bourgeois tastes, nevertheless perpetuate the views that study of the interior of the human body can only be explored by invasive or violent acts and that our relationship with death in the 20th century is essentially a pathological one.

For Ian Breakwell, however, death is not denied or banished but accepted in all its guises – from the tragic to the humorous. It is not his intention to shock with macabre imagery but to confront the viewer with his or her own mortality. Over a period of 30 years, Breakwell has made self-portraits which chronicle his changing facial appearance from childhood to anticipated old age, as in the 1985 photo-triptych *The Mask* in which prosthetic make-up was used to visualise his face as it might have been in the year 2000. During the last few years, Breakwell's concern with the theme of mortality has particularly been focused on a sociocultural interpretation of the "Dance of Death". Amongst the numerous original artworks produced, three major works have been developed as a result of Breakwell's researches into the theme: *The Rose, Deathrap* and *Death Masks*.

# The Rose

Based directly on the theme of the "Dance of Death", *The Rose* is an audiovisual artwork that features an illuminated light-box in the form of a rose window filled with hundreds of interlocked skeletons, with personal stereo headset sound by the composer Ron Geesin. The work is designed specifically for solo viewing and listening in a small study room; visitors are invited to sit, look, and listen to *The Rose* for as long as they wish, with the same quiet contemplation they would devote to the study of a book.

Rose windows have their origins in mandalas, circular labyrinths and the radial designs of Early Christian and Byzantine church domes. By the 10th century the spoked wheel window was common, often as a Wheel of Fortune with figures dragged around the perimeter to their death, illustrating the temporary nature of worldly success in an ungodly life. The wheel window evolved into the classic rose window that drew attention away from the circumference and focused on the centre through which all opposites are reconciled within a surrounding circular unity.

Often the circle is architecturally contained within a square, symbolising the interdependence of the finite and the infinite. Geometric perfection is intended to express divine proportion and order. In its final flamboyant phase the rose window transformed into a radiating tracery of curvilinear flames. Symbolically, the rose signifies both human and divine love; passionate love but also love beyond passion. In Dante's *Divine Comedy*, Paradise is constructed as a rose. The rose window also symbolises the sun (the source of all light) and the star (the guiding light in the struggle of the spirit against the forces of darkness).

The visual form of Breakwell's *The Rose* is indeed a circle within a square, based upon the structure of the rose window in Durham Cathedral where Ian Breakwell was Artist-in-Residence during 1994–95. Breakwell contradicts the geometric symmetry of the rose, symbol of the perfect wholeness of the world, by superimposing its design onto a whirling tango of death. This paradox refers back to the rose window's medieval forerunner, the Wheel of Fortune window. Instead of the myriad colours of stained glass, *The Rose* is saturated with one intense red hue, referring to the colour of the flower, to blood, and to the evocation of flames within late rose windows. The taped sound of *The Rose* is composed from three sources: William Blake's poem *The Sick Rose* (spoken by Ian Breakwell), with its symbolism of the parasitic corruption of beauty and order; the game song "Ring-A-Rosey" (sung by school children), often thought to have its roots in the Black Death; and a tolling bell, also associated with the plague as a call for the dead to be brought out to be buried.

# Deathrap

Ian Breakwell has interpreted the allegorical theme and skeletal imagery of the "Dance of Death" in a variety of new guises. Works made encompass photo-text sequences, photomontage, digitally manipulated inkjet prints and Duratrans light-box installation. In its original form, *Deathrap* was a series of Xerox collages with calligraphic caption sequential text. In the later tape-slide version, pliable toy skeletons, manipulated in a photocopying machine, have then been silhouetted as hundreds of skeletal paper cut-outs in a manner similar to that used in Mexican Day of the Dead *papeles picados*. The result is a "cinematic", five-minute animation called *Deathrap*, in which the "Dance of Death" is paradoxically portrayed as the all-action climax of the carnival of life. The animated, life-size images of skeletal dancers move to sync-pulsed music composed by Ron Geesin. Chronologically, two skeletons meet and enjoin in a slow jive, which develops into a tap dance, which turns into an acrobatic break dance where gradually more and more skeletons join in, as the rhythmically percussive music gathers pace until the screen is filled with scores of writhing, interlocked skeletons raving at frenetic speed to a pulsing climax of sound.

A recurring characteristic of the cultural history of the "Dance of Death" relates to the fact that the skeletal figures of Death are often portrayed as being livelier than the living. This feature is clearly represented in *Deathrap* where the skeletons take over the dance floor and dance only with themselves. The theme of the animated skeleton as an entertainment feature has a long history. As Felicity Sparrow[8] has shown in her study of pre-cinematic audiovisual entertainment, phantasmagoria, magic lantern acts and stage illusions were commonplace in the early 19th century and these often featured dancing skeletons, which inspired terror and awe in their audiences. In recent times, the comedic effects of Melies and Walt Disney and the world of healthcare advertising have used similar imagery.

Combining the thrill of the macabre with the humour of impossible contortions as fleshless bones move on their own, the imagery is universal and does not need dialogue for audiences to respond. The visual style of *Deathrap* draws on this cinematic tradition: the conjoined skeletal figures are also suggestive of X-rays and sometimes of fetal scans. They can be ambiguously interpreted as dancing or struggling or even as being entangled in extreme sexual acrobatics. Whatever it is, they are doing it to the liveliest mix of images and music. It almost seems as if Breakwell is inviting the viewers to rise from their seats and join in "The Dance"!

## Death Masks

The portrayal of an inanimate face that is paradoxically expressive is developed in the series of *Death Masks* that Breakwell has made using thermal imaging cameras. Thermography is normally used for medical diagnosis (for example, for detecting tumours, vascular defects, inflammation, and arthritis). It provides a picture of the heat structure of the human body by reading the infrared radiation so that the final computer-generated image translates what is invisible to the naked eye into a visible language. A similar process underlies Breakwell's images and indeed informs the transition from life to death (from the visible to the invisible). Breakwell manipulates a variety of facemasks to trap heat from the head and to record fluctuations using inhaled and exhaled breath from the nose and mouth. Such manipulations are combined with exaggerated facial muscle movement. To the human eye the monochrome mask remains impassive, but the thermal camera sees through the mask to the colourful turmoil it hides.[9]

*Body Mask* is a companion piece to *Death Mask*. This features a full-body radiograph of Ian Breakwell, accompanied by a text on the theme of bruising. The work hints at death and not merely from the use of the anatomical imagery nor from the self-portrait's allusion to a *memento mori*. Both the text and the folded, facedown body image suggest a violent death. Furthermore, there are psychological elements at play. The bruising is not necessarily physical and the very title *Body Mask*, together with the reference to the skeleton within the depth of the body, also implies that to hide behind a mask need not involve an external deceit but an internal (psychological) deceit. The denying of death to oneself is just such a deceit.

The "Dance of Death" project is, of course, an artistic and scientific collaboration undertaken by a well-established artist and medical/scientific staff. However, such projects can be undertaken by the medical student, given the recent development of special study modules in the medical curriculum where students are free to take options which interest them and thereby to go beyond the defined core curriculum. It is, however, necessary for the curriculum organisers and medical teachers to acknowledge the importance of, and be aware of, the opportunities for introducing the creative arts into the curriculum. Other examples of artistic involvement can be found in the practice of having life drawing classes for a mixed group of art students and medical students, overseen by art teachers, professional artists and basic medical scientists. In addition, incorporation of modules on the history of medicine would be beneficial. To introduce the creative arts into medical courses the curriculum planners need to be aware of two problems.

First, there is the danger of increasing factual and intellectual overload. This cannot be justified if it involves the diminution of important, core scientific aspects of the curriculum. Indeed, there will be no progress (and potentially only conflict) if it is seen that the introduction of the humanities continues to demean science and shifts medicine further from being an applied science to an applied social science! Second, students should not be over-examined in such material, but should be allowed to develop their creative skills through being highly motivated and by the device of awarding students further progression onto the course via the notion of "successful completion" and not examination grading. Given the constraints of time and the need to continue to teach core topics within existing medical courses, perhaps the best way forward for introducing the humanities into medicine is just to abandon entrance to medical school straight from secondary school with scientific subject awards.

Perhaps more benefit to the profession (and to patients) will arise by having postgraduate entry to medicine, accepting that some of the medical students will have progressed through arts and humanities degrees. The cynic will of course raise the question: what, in terms of entrance to medical school, is so special about art and artists? Why should we not be conferring special privileges on sportsmen, on comedians, and on philosophers?! Of course, all of these (and more) add value to the medical profession. What we need to convince the cynic is that they add value to the patients' treatments and prognoses!

Finally, I am bound to record that my experience on the "Dance of Death" project has convinced me that, whilst there is undoubted benefit to medicine in incorporating the creative arts, there is also a considerable benefit to the creative arts from an understanding, and appreciation, of the medical sciences.

## References and notes

1    Illich I. *Limits to Medicine. Medical Nemesis: the expropriation of health.* Harmondsworth: Penguin Books, 1976.
2    Gorer G. The pornography of death. In: *Death, Grief and Mourning in Contemporary Britain.* London: Cresset Press, 1965.
3    Aries P. *The Hour of Our Death.* New York: Alfred A Knopf, 1981.
4    Benjamin W. *Illuminations.* New York: Schocken Books, 1969.
5    Townsend C. *Vile Bodies.* Munich/New York: Prestel, 1998.
6    Gott T (ed.). *Don't Leave Me This Way: art in the age of AIDS.* Canberra: National Gallery of Australia, 1994.
7    Petherbridge D, Jordanova L. *The Quick and the Dead.* London: South Bank Centre, 1997.
8    Sparrow F. *Through the Large Glass.* London: London College of Printing, 1997.
9    Sawday J. *The Body Emblazoned.* London: Routledge, 1995.

# 11

# United in grief: monuments and memories of the Great War

Angela Gaffney[1]

For thousands of men in France and Flanders the chill, still greyness of a November morning in 1918 was unremarkable. But this day would be different. A signal was issued that at 11.00 am an Armistice would come into effect which officially ceased hostilities. By the time the guns finally fell silent, an estimated nine million men had lost their lives in the Great War and over 700 000 of these were British servicemen.[2] Adrian Gregory has suggested that an estimated three million Britons lost a close relative in the Great War although, as he points out, "This figure represents only the 'primary bereaved' (parents, siblings, widows, and orphans). In addition, the 'secondary bereaved' ought to be considered, those who lost a cousin, uncle, son-in-law, a colleague, a friend or a neighbour".[3] The loss of life on this scale ensured that bereavement became a shared experience throughout Britain as individuals and communities attempted to come to terms with their grief. Memorials were erected during the war, often in the form of street shrines which initially served to honour those men who had volunteered for service and some of these were later incorporated into war memorials.[4] The decade following the Armistice, however, witnessed a determination to provide a lasting tribute to those who had died. War memorials in virtually every town and village provide testimony to the need felt by society in the postwar years to commemorate the dead.

Casualty lists published in British newspapers throughout the war gave daily notice of the catastrophic impact on a society that in many ways was simply not prepared for death. Improvements in medical care combined with decreased infant mortality rates in the late 19th and early 20th centuries had created the expectation that children would outlive their parents.[5] Writing in 1915, Freud noted that the war was "bound to sweep away this conventional treatment of death. Death will no longer be denied; we are forced to believe in it. People really die; and no longer one by one, but many, often tens of thousands, in a single day. And death is no longer a chance event."[6]

The physical effect of mechanised warfare was compounded by the decision taken in 1915 to ban repatriation of bodies from the battlefield. This was taken on the grounds of hygiene and also "on account of the difficulties of treating impartially the claims advanced by persons of different social standing."[7] It appeared that the formalities of burial were being taken over by officialdom in the form of the Imperial War Graves Commission whose policy was guided by the principle of equality of sacrifice and therefore equality of commemoration. To the bereaved relatives this appeared a remote and bureaucratic process into which they had little input apart from choosing a personal inscription for the official headstone. Pilgrimages were organised to the battlefields in the decade after the war to enable relatives of the dead to visit either an individual grave or a memorial.[8] For many bereaved families, however, the ability to travel abroad, even at a low price, would have been extremely limited. The decade following the war witnessed high unemployment in areas of Britain and foreign travel was simply not an option.

With so many people unable to visit, if not the grave then the assumed site of death, the mass emotional outburst of the British public that surrounded the erection of the Cenotaph in London in 1919 was perhaps understandable. It had been built as a temporary structure for the Peace Day Celebrations to provide a saluting point for the Allied troops at the Victory March in July 1919 to celebrate the signing of the Treaty of Versailles. In the weeks after Peace Day increasing numbers of people came to lay wreaths at the Cenotaph. It was claimed that by the first week of August 1919 half a million people visited the monument as it became a place of pilgrimage and mourning. Pressure grew for the temporary structure to be made permanent and on Armistice Day 1920 the structure that we see today was unveiled as part of the same ceremony to bury an Unknown Warrior in Westminster Abbey.[9] The strength of the public reaction was testament to the overwhelming need for a permanent, tangible reminder of the dead within local communities.

Memorials to those killed in the Great War were erected in communities which had already suffered tragedy, often on a far greater scale than that inflicted by the Great War. In October 1913 the village of Senghennydd in the Aber Valley in south Wales endured the worst accident in British mining history when an explosion underground at the Universal Colliery killed 439 men and boys.[10] This occurred just 12 years after a similar explosion claimed 79 lives at the same pit. The impressive clock tower that stands in the centre of the square in Senghennydd records not the mining accident of 1913 but the 63 men from the village who were killed in the Great War. The memorial was unveiled in 1921, only eight years after the pit tragedy which had claimed so many more local lives than the war but until recently there was no official memorial to the 1913 disaster.[11] Yet war is not dissimilar to mining accidents; both can cut a swathe through the male population of a community, leaving desolation and often deprivation in their wake. Death underground was a harsh but unavoidable fact of life in industrial Wales, but the proliferation of war memorials in such communities cannot be attributed solely to pride in local sacrifice for a higher cause.

Accounts of rescue operations following pit explosions include stories of great courage and immense danger for those involved in the struggle for survivors. A similar sense of urgency is apparent even when all hope of life has faded as it becomes no less important to retrieve bodies from the mine wherever possible. This was evident in the aftermath of the Senghennydd explosion in 1913, when the urgency was fuelled by "strongly held feelings about the significance of a proper burial and of a horror, common in all coalfields, of leaving bodies in a mine."[12]

Death and burial on the battlefield, however, denied those left behind the opportunity to participate in the funeral ritual, a process accepted to be an intrinsic and integral part of the grieving process by helping the bereaved to face the reality of death. Raymond Firth has written that a "funeral rite is a social rite par excellence. Its ostensible object is the dead person, but it benefits not the dead, but the living... As anthropologists have so often stressed, it is those who are left behind – the kinsfolk, the neighbours, and other members of the community – for whom the ritual is really performed".[13] Firth maintains that the ritual of a funeral provides an opportunity for the "resolution of uncertainties" for the immediate kin. The keenness of grief may have become blunted, but acceptance of death is still emotionally difficult and a funeral rite provides a cathartic mechanism for a public display of grief. The bereaved families of the Great War simply did not have a visual object for their grief and the personal inscriptions chosen for the headstones in the war cemeteries often reflected the pain that this caused. Private James Wyper of the King's Own Scottish Borderers was killed in September 1916 aged 24 and is buried in Abbeville Communal Cemetery in northern France; the inscription at the foot of his headstone reads: "Too far away thy grave to see but not too far to think of thee".

Erecting a war memorial, the ritual involved in the subsequent unveiling ceremonies and the position of the memorial invariably at the centre of a community both literally and figuratively, acted as an emotional catharsis enabling the bereaved to begin to accept the death of a loved one and to contemplate moving forward once more. In this context, commemoration of the individual was extremely important, as the local memorial became the surrogate grave providing an essential focus for individual and collective grief. As many families were denied the opportunity to bury their loved ones, they sought emotional consolation from the ritual and ceremonies of local war memorials.

The legacy of loss and emotional trauma is marked today by the crosses, cenotaphs, obelisks, figurative sculpture, and other forms of war memorial which can be found throughout Britain. Such memorials remain as potent evidence both of the catastrophe of the Great War and of the challenges faced by those seeking to commemorate the fallen. Exhibitions of war memorial designs were held at the Victoria and Albert Museum and the Royal Academy of Arts in 1919, but there was no "official" central direction or funding for commemoration. Even the collection of names to be inscribed on memorials was undertaken on a local and voluntary basis, unlike in France where "the names of those officially deemed to have died for the nation were supplied from Paris".[14] War memorials were a spontaneous act of a community whether village, town or city; people wanted them, they were not imposed on communities. Most memorials were funded by public subscription and organised by local committees chosen to reflect the structure of society but which inevitably also reflected the social hierarchy of a community.[15] Local councillors, schoolmasters, industrialists, and landowners were amongst the usual members of such committees, primarily due to their position within the community and most were, at this time, invariably male. Of course, with so many families affected either directly or indirectly by the war, the probability must be that most members of memorial committees would have a claim to be counted amongst the "bereaved". It seems more likely that women were on memorial committees because they were already engaged in similar work. The minutes of the War Memorial Committee in Barry, south Wales, specifically refer to co-opting on to the committee four representatives of "women's organisations in the district".[16]

It appears that throughout Britain the need to commemorate the fallen was not a matter for public debate although the site, size, and cost of memorials stimulated much discussion. It was the form of memorial that usually caused most controversy within communities, with heated debate often taking place over whether a community should opt for a utilitarian or sacred memorial and whether a memorial should serve the living or honour the dead. The potential loss of meaning attached to a utilitarian memorial was often cited in opposing this form of commemoration.[17] If buildings such as halls or hospitals were interpreted as minimising the spirit of those to whom they were erected, they could serve to increase the burden of mourning rather than providing emotional solace.

Memorials in the form of figurative sculpture were particularly important in the grieving process. Catherine Moriarty has written of the figurative sculpture of the Great War providing "one symbolic body which replaced the many absent, fragmented corpses which were, at this time, still being salvaged from the battlefields, reinterred and, if possible identified. Never before had a single body represented so many who had 'passed out of the sight of men.' The dead's very absence facilitated the process of idealisation, of whom they had been as people and the circumstances of their death".[18] By providing a constant visible reminder of the dead, the meaning of a monument was unambiguous and enduring.

Ironically it was often those most affected by the war who were marginalised by the commemorative process, most notably the bereaved families who had a negligible input into the "official" commemoration of the nation's dead. At a national level there were no women present at the first meeting of the Imperial War Graves Commissioners in November 1917 although unsuccessful attempts had been made by various women's organisations to gain representation.[19] It was unusual for women to be represented as wives, mothers or sisters on local war memorial committees. As a group the bereaved families were rarely either considered or consulted in the commemorative process although becoming involved in what was essentially a business arrangement may have been neither appropriate nor practical after the war. Many women may have chosen voluntarily not to participate in memorial committees as they struggled both to come to terms with their loss and to cope with the realities of postwar life. Eleanor Cain became a wife and widow within 11 months, losing her husband, baby, and brother; she "felt like lying down and giving up altogether" whilst Kitty Eckersley heard the news of her husband's death when she was seven months pregnant. She recalled that she did not want to live because "the world had come to an end then for me because I'd lost all that I loved".[20]

It is clear that the "bereaved" extended beyond the immediate family group and included men as well as women yet there is an implicit assumption in reports of the commemorative process that the bereaved are women. It was usually in their role as grieving mothers that women participated in the commemorative process by unveiling local memorials, but their visual image was deemed sufficient as on such occasions the women usually did not address the crowd attending the ceremony.[21] Occasionally, a bereaved father performed the unveiling ceremony, as at Bala in north Wales where Mr John Davies unveiled the local memorial, but did not address the crowd. Mr Davies had lost two sons in the war. In Penarth, south Wales, Mr G Hoult, who had lost three sons in the war, was due to share the unveiling with two bereaved mothers, but a few days before the ceremony he decided not to take part. The local paper reported that "he preferred not to undergo the trying ordeal".[22]

The unveiling ceremony itself was frequently described in local newspapers as the "highlight of the year" and was reported in great detail. As the war memorial could be viewed as a surrogate grave, the unveiling ceremony took on the guise of a funeral service under the watchful eye of the church. A religious presence, usually in the form of prayers, blessings, and dedication, was an intrinsic part of ceremonies whether the memorial was sacred or utilitarian in nature and these were often combined with extracts from the burial service.[23] Yet religion was not always able to offer an effective panacea to the grief experienced by so many families in the postwar years which prompted some to look elsewhere for consolation or to make attempts to contact their loved ones. Spiritualism witnessed an unprecedented growth in popularity during and after the war as the bereaved attempted to come to terms with their loss and it is clear that while the Christian message played an important role in the amelioration of grief for some, it proved insubstantial and inadequate for others.[24]

Despite the apparent exclusion of the bereaved from the

commemorative process, whether self-inflicted or not, the many small ceremonies held to unveil memorials in schools, churches, and workplaces throughout Britain provided an immediate outlet for grief. In July 1921 a tablet was unveiled at Cadoxton Boys" School in Barry in memory of 68 old boys who died in the Great War and the ceremony was punctuated by "the sobbing of grief-stricken mothers".[25] Larger, civic memorials with elaborate unveiling ceremonies may have seemed remote both physically and psychologically to many bereaved families and the importance and immediacy of local commemoration is apparent as usually little interest was shown in more comprehensive projects. Local commemoration provided those left behind with an immediate, daily reminder of the sacrifice made by husbands, fathers, lovers, sons or brothers. It was a very public affirmation of community, with the memorial itself acting as a "marker" by signifying its exclusivity and uniqueness. It proclaimed a local contribution to the war not only by mourning the loss of its young men, but by making a clear statement that these were "our" young men echoing Edna Longley's comment that "Commemorations are as selective as sympathies. They honour *our* dead, not your dead".[26]

It is clear that the invocation of civic pride played a prominent role in the commemoration process as newspapers frequently sought to compare communities still without a memorial to those who had "done the right thing" or were in the process of doing so. The appeal to civic pride was often combined with the implicit accusation that the absence of a memorial, or a movement to build one, displayed a lack of honour and respect for the dead. Newspaper comments were acerbic in their condemnation of local indifference to sacrifices made in the Great War.

At one time there was much talk of Aberdare going to do a lot for the survivors of the Great War and also for the memory of those who fell. We were going to erect a cenotaph and a new memorial hall and ever so many other monuments of gratitude and appreciation. But all those elaborate schemes have gone the way of the best laid schemes of mice and men and the abstract homes fit for heroes to live in. "Lest we forget" indeed! We have forgotten already. Buying poppies is far cheaper than building halls and houses.[27]

At times the commemoration process itself may have served to alienate and marginalise the bereaved. In the small village of

Crickhowell, a succession of parish council meetings in late 1918 and early 1919 was held to make arrangements for returning soldiers and prisoners of war. It was decided to present a silver medallion and ten-shilling note to each returning soldier and to the next of kin of deceased officers and men. This took place at a church parade held in the town square in September 1919. A parish meeting later in September resolved to recall the medallions given to the next of kin of the deceased and that the words "Welcome Home" be crossed off and "For King and Country" inscribed in their place.[28]

The Second World War and subsequent conflicts prompted a new era of commemoration although names of the fallen have often been added to existing memorials. Heated debate took place in America over the proposed Vietnam Memorial. The very real problem in reaching a consensus view on the meaning of American involvement in Vietnam was a major factor in the arguments surrounding the controversial sculpture but the role of the traditional war memorial in the healing process was acknowledged. Lisa Capps conducted interviews with visitors to the memorial, including veterans, relatives of the dead, citizens, and tourists, and concluded that: "War creates wounds – figuratively as well as literally. . . These wounds are acknowledged as the war is discussed and clarified, and as we work toward understanding individual losses, personal tragedies in the light of positive national significance. Healing occurs as we bestow meaning upon the war experience. War memorials both signify and promote this process".[29]

The desire for public commemoration is as potent in the opening year of the new century as it was nearly 100 years ago. Individual and collective loss under tragic circumstances is usually marked by impromptu spontaneous commemoration followed in due course by a more permanent memorial. The role of the media is crucial as their unquenchable thirst for "human-life" drama often results in high-profile but limited publicity until the next crisis diverts public attention and sympathy. The fear of forgetting has become an integral part of remembrance as "lest we forget" becomes almost an admonition to society. The location of a memorial remains a crucial element in the commemorative process. Unlike regional and national memorials, local commemoration is relevant, accessible and provides a permanent, daily reminder of collective and individual loss. War memorials in particular remain in our urban and rural landscape as markers of local identity and civic pride yet also reveal the individual pain of bereavement, emphasising their central role in the grieving process. Jay Winter has written:

How healing occurs, and what quietens embitterment and alleviates despair can never be fully known. But not to ask the question, not to try to place the history of war memorials within the history of bereavement, a history we all share in our private lives, is both to impoverish the study of history and to evade our responsibility as historians. For we must attend to the faces and feelings of those who were bereft, and who made the pilgrimages to these sites of memory, large and small, in order to begin to understand how men and women tried to cope with one of the signal catastrophes of our century.[30]

# References and notes

1   Material for this chapter was drawn from my PhD thesis: Poppies on the up-platform: Commemoration of the Great War in Wales (University of Wales Press, Cardiff, 1996) and from my book *Aftermath: Remembering the Great War in Wales* (University of Wales Press, Cardiff, 1998).

2   Winter JM. *The Great War and the British people*. London: Macmillan, 1986: 71.

3   Gregory A. *The Silence of Memory*. Oxford: Berg, 1994: 19.

4   See, for example, Goodman A. *The Street Memorials of St Albans Abbey Parish*. St Albans: St Albans and Hertfordshire Architectural and Archaeological Society, 1987.

5   See Cannadine D. War and death, grief and mourning in modern Britain. In: Whaley J (ed.). *Mirrors of Mortality: studies in the social history of death*. London: Europa Publications, 1981: 217. See also Tarlow S. *Bereavement and Commemoration: an archaeology of mortality*. Oxford: Blackwell, 1999.

6   Freud S. Thoughts for the times on war and death. In: Strachey J, Freud A (eds). *The Standard Edition of the Complete Psychological Works of Sigmund Freud*, vol.XIV, 1914–1916. London: Hogarth Press, 1957: 291.

7   Longworth P. *The Unending Vigil. A History of the Commonwealth War Graves Commission 1917–1984*. London: Leo Cooper, 1985: 14. Similar debates took place in America where almost 70% of families opted for repatriation of bodies. In 1919 some of those urging repatriation formed the "Bring Back the Dead League". For the remainder of the dead, the US government established a number of permanent cemeteries in France, Belgium and England. See Piehler GK. In: Gillis JR (ed.). The war dead and the Gold Star: American commemoration of the First World War. *Commemorations: The politics of national identity*. Princeton: Princeton University Press, 1994.

8   Lloyd DW. *Battlefield Tourism. Pilgrimage and the Commemoration of the Great War in Britain, Australia and Canada, 1919–1939*. Oxford: Berg, 1998. See also Walter T. War grave pilgrimage. In: Reader I, Walter T (eds). *Pilgrimage in Popular Culture*. London: Macmillan, 1993: 63–91.

9   For accounts of the building of the Cenotaph, see Homberger E. The story of the Cenotaph. *Times Literary Supplement* 1976; 12 November: 1429–30; Greenberg A. Lutyens" Cenotaph. *J Soc Architectural Historians* 1989; **48**: 5–23; Curtis P. The Whitehall Cenotaph: an accidental monument. *Imperial War Museum Rev* 1994; **9**: 31–41.

10  For details of the Senghennydd explosion, see Brown JH. *The Valley of the Shadow*. Port Talbot: Alun Books, 1981; Williams R, Jones D. *The Cruel Inheritance*. Pontypool: Village Publishing, 1990: 74–82; Lieven M. *Senghennydd: the Universal pit village, 1890–1930*. Llandysul: Gomer Press, 1994: 215–68.

11  A memorial to the victims of the 1901 and 1913 disaster was unveiled in Senghennydd in October 1981.

12  Lieven M[10], 236. An explosion at Gresford Colliery in north Wales in 1934 claimed the lives of 261 miners but due to the dangerous conditions it was not possible to retrieve all the bodies from the mine. See Laidlaw R. The Gresford disaster in popular memory. *Llafur* 1995; **VI**: 123–46.

13  Firth R. *Elements of Social Organization*. London: CA Watts, 1951: 63. See also Huppauf B. War and death: the experience of the First World War. In: Crouch M, Huppauf B (eds). *Essays on Mortality*. Sydney: University of New South Wales, 1985.

14  Inglis KS. War memorials: ten questions for historians. *Guerres Mondiales et Conflits Contemporains* 1992; CLXVII: 5–21.

15  Alex King has written in detail on the composition and power structures within local memorial committees. King A. *Memorials of the Great War in Britain. The Symbolism and Politics of Remembrance*. Oxford: Berg, 1998.

16  Barry Urban District Council 12 December 1921. Report of a meeting of Barry War Memorial Committee held on 24 November 1921.

17  Curl JS. *A Celebration of Death*. London: Constable, 1980.

18  Moriarty C. The absent dead and figurative First World War memorials. *Trans Ancient Monuments Soc* 1995; **39**: 7–40.

19  Longworth P[7], 29.

20  Interviews taken from the Imperial War Museum Sound Archive.

21  Mothers who had lost sons in the war unveiled memorials in Wales at Brecon, Dolgellau, Kidwelly, Llanfairpwllgwyngyll, Mumbles and Penarth.

22  *Penarth News*; 1924; 13 November.

23  See Moriarty C. Christian iconography and First World War memorials. *Imperial War Museum Rev* 1992; **6**: 63–75. For memorials as religious symbols, see Davies J. War Memorials. In: Clark D (ed.). *The Sociology of Death*. Oxford: Blackwell, 1993.

24  A full account of this phenomenon is given by Winter JM. *Sites of Memory, Sites of Mourning: the Great War in European cultural history*. Cambridge: Cambridge University Press, 1995: 54–77. See also Hazelgrove JM. *Spiritualism and British Society Between the Wars*. Manchester: Manchester University Press, 2000.

25  *Barry Dock News* 1921; 22 July.

26  Longley E. The Rising, the Somme and Irish Memory. In: Ni Dhonnchadha M, Morgan T (eds). *Revising the Rising*. Londonderry: Field Day, 1991.

27  *Aberdare Leader* 1921; 19 November.

28  See minutes of Crickhowell Parish Council, especially 18 September 1919.

29  Capps LM. The memorial as symbol and agent of healing. In: Capps W (ed.). *The Vietnam Reader*. London: Routledge, 1991: 272.

30  Winter[24], 116.

# 12

# Why medical humanities now?

Jane Macnaughton

## Context: Why medical humanities now?

There seems to have been an epidemic of arts and humanities courses breaking out in medical schools all over the country. Newcastle, Nottingham, Royal Free and UCL, Guy's, King's and St Thomas', Aberdeen, Cardiff, Leeds and others are running special study modules for students with titles such as "Poetry, Novels and Medicine" (Newcastle) and "Visualising/Modifying the Body in Art and Medicine" (Guy's, King's and St Thomas'). These courses are proving very popular and students compete for places on them. There is also growing interest in the humanities in postgraduate medical education. A course has been run in Ripon for general practice trainers to encourage them to use the arts and humanities in the training of their GP registrars and the Swansea MA in Medical Humanities is now well established.

In tandem with these developments in medical education is the growth of interest and activity in the arts as therapy. There are three ways in which the arts are being used for therapeutic purposes. First, there are the arts therapies proper where visual art, music, dance, and creative writing are being used by specifically trained practitioners working with groups or individuals who have an illness or disability. Music and art therapy are officially recognised as professions allied to medicine and have professional status and a recognised training.[1] Also working in healthcare contexts are artists or healthcare professionals who are using various art forms in their treatment of patients. This forms the second group who are not specifically trained in art therapy but who are developing expertise through practice. The third way in which the arts are being used is for community development and health. In this context health promoters, local arts organisations and individual artists are working not in healthcare contexts with people who are ill but with communities or groups within communities which have high deprivation and are regarded as socially excluded.

It is this last group of activities which has helped to thrust the arts and health movement into the limelight, as social exclusion is now regarded as a major determinant of ill health[2] and is recognised as such by the government who are interested in anything that may contribute to tackling it.[3] There is, therefore, a political imperative to encourage the development of community arts and health projects and the government has even made mention of the importance of these activities in the White Paper on health, *Saving Lives: our Healthier Nation*, commenting that "participation in the arts and sport can promote social cohesion by building strong social networks".[4]

## Medical humanities and arts and health: a relationship

But is there a similar imperative to develop arts and humanities within medical education? The two movements seem on the face of it to be related as they both deal with applications of the arts in health and medicine. However, the arts and health movement is dedicated to therapy whereas the medical humanities movement is concerned first, with the educational development of the health practitioner and second, with the critical examination of the nature of healthcare and medical practice and its evidence base. The former movement is a community and health-related activity, while the latter has grown up within universities, largely within medical schools. The origins of both movements can, however, be traced to some common roots: changing views of the determinants of health and related changes in society's view of biomedical medicine and of doctors who practise it. Let us examine these common roots.

The current New Labour government in the UK has explicitly acknowledged the fact that "the social, economic and environmental factors tending towards poor health are potent" and that inequalities in health between richer and poorer are a widespread problem.[4] This acceptance has committed the government and the health services to examine ways of tackling the determinants of health inequalities. Until now the NHS has focused its attention on tackling the health of the individual but, as Richard Wilkinson says in his seminal book on the social determinants of health:

...the important factors which make some societies healthier than others may be quite different from those which differ between healthy and unhealthy individuals within the same society.[5]

Those important factors, according to Wilkinson, include the extent of economic and social equality within the society and the extent to which people feel they have control over their lives. The problem is not so much to do with absolute levels of poverty but rather the large gradients between the haves and the have nots. These issues are not ones which we would expect to be the concern of health services. Rather they are the concern of governments and welfare agencies. But as they are now being recognised as important for health, doctors must be aware of the problem of societal inequality and consider ways of tackling the lack of control that it produces.

This new social and economic view of the origins of health problems is a challenge to the pervasive biomedical approach to medicine in the UK and most western societies. It is a challenge to doctors to promote a new way of working and, in consequence, to encourage a change to the way in which future doctors are educated. The arts and health movement is responding to this changing view by using the arts to promote greater social cohesion and involvement. There is evidence that community arts and health projects are having this effect. A recent report published by the independent research organisation Comedia found that participation in the arts can increase people's confidence and sense of self-worth, extend involvement in social activity and encourage adults to take up education and training experiences.[6] What is now required from doctors and from doctors in training is a wider perception of what influences health and a broader conceptual understanding of the basis of health inequalities and how these cause ill health. In turn this should encourage doctors to develop a bigger toolkit for tackling health problems.

This brings us back to the connection between arts and health and medical humanities. The arts and health movement is a response to the need to tackle social exclusion through community involvement with the arts. The medical humanities movement may be seen as an attempt to extend the range of doctors beyond biomedicine in two ways. First, by extending the scope of medical education beyond biomedicine, doctors can access a whole new range of concepts for understanding the variety of contexts in which health-improving activities can take place, the varied types of evidence relevant to different aspects of the medical consultation and, indeed, for understanding health itself in its varied meanings for different people. Second, the traditional and rapidly expanding technical expertise of biomedicine can be given a humane basis. I will go on to illustrate these roles of medical humanities later in the chapter.

## Educational context

As well as having a relationship to the parallel arts and health movement, the medical humanities movement has arisen against the background of changes in the educational context. In the past ethics was the subject that both brought humanities back into the context of medical education and also brought academics such as philosophers and theologians into medical education. But now, as part of the need to widen the basis for medical expertise, there is a move to suggest that the teaching of ethics is too narrow a field to take in the range of moral and personal difficulties that may affect clinical decision making. This point is taken up by Robin Downie in the *Journal of Medical Ethics*.[7] In a commentary on a poem, Downie argues that most of what has been traditionally taught via undergraduate courses on medical ethics can be better taught in the richer context of the medical humanities. This richer context can provide a wide non-medical perspective on problems in medical ethics and assist with the "consciousness-raising" aspects of ethics. The point here is while medical ethics tends to concentrate on what are called "dilemmas", many of the criticisms of doctors derive from the fact that they have a manner which patients find arrogant or they can write letters unaware of the impact these might have on their patients. The humanities can hold up a mirror to ourselves, which the more theoretical approach of philosophical medical ethics cannot do. In short, ethics is too narrow a field to take in the understanding of the full range of qualities that the physician must have in order to practise humanely. This was understood in the 18th century when Professor John Gregory was lecturing to his students at the University of Edinburgh on the moral qualities which he thought the physician should have. Chief of these, he says, is humanity, which he describes in this way.

... that sensibility of heart which makes us feel for the distresses of our fellow creatures, and which of consequence incites us in the most powerful manner to relieve them.[8]

– a simple but very beautiful characterisation of this quality. He goes on to note the other qualities which should be possessed by the humane physician, which are "good humour", "gentleness" and even "flexibility", arguing that if a doctor is too authoritarian with his patients he will not encourage compliance. This is what we might nowadays call an encouragement to "patient-centred" care. It may be that the umbrella discipline for ethics in the future may be medical humanities which will allow the fuller consideration of all these qualities in the developing doctor.

The expansion in the number of medical schools and the need to train more doctors are also having an effect on admission criteria. Wider access to prospective students who have been educated in other disciplines, including the arts, is being encouraged. Teaching methods within medical schools are diversifying from the standard method of information giving in large group lectures to increasing focus on small group teaching and problem-based learning. These encourage the students to think for themselves and to be more critically aware of what they are being taught, very much the attributes of the humanely educated arts student.

Above all, the undergraduate medical educational context has changed through the efforts of the General Medical Council. In 1993 they recognised that medical education needed a radical rethink and in their report *Tomorrow's Doctors*[9] they recommended a greater focus on education, as opposed to training, in the undergraduate degree. The good doctor, as the GMC suggest, must be an educated doctor and this is one of the major areas where arts and humanities subjects might make a contribution.[7]

The medical humanities movement has, therefore, grown up with the arts and health movement and has some common roots and some distinctive roots. Granted the need for a new approach to medical education, how do the humanities contribute to the creation of this humane expert with a broad conception of the doctor's toolkit?

# Justifications

There are two main ways in which humanities subjects might be relevant to medicine. One, often discussed, is that the humanities play a primarily *instrumental* role in the education of future doctors.[10] Works of literature in particular may help to introduce students to problematic life situations with which they may be unfamiliar. Imaginative identification with the characters involved will allow them at least vicarious experience of these problems before having to deal with them as doctors in a clinical situation. Students may also learn useful skills from the humanities, such as good (and poor) oral communication from drama or the skill of analysis and argument (as we shall later see) from philosophy. But it would be to devalue the arts and the humanities to suggest that they should be seen merely as a means to an end, even in the context of professional or vocational education.[11] Art, literature, drama, and music, in all their many forms, are expressions of human creativity; they reflect human joy and sorrow, and human celebration and reflection. Part of what it is to be a complete human being is to participate in some form of artistic activity, either as spectator, reader or viewer. Understanding this will help doctors to remember the purpose of their own art: to enable people to participate fully in life unhampered as far as possible by illness or disability.

The humanities, therefore, have a second, *non-instrumental* role in the education of doctors. They do not merely have a *usefulness* in contributing to the development of ends other than themselves: they also have an intrinsic *value* in their own right and as such are essential components of the educated mind. As Downie puts it, "Along with an understanding of the sciences they constitute what it means to be 'educated' as distinct from simply 'trained'".[7]

There is not, of course, a straightforward distinction between the instrumental and the non-instrumental uses of the humanities. For example, I have suggested that the understanding of the human condition which may come from literature is an instrumental use, but it is also part of a general educative process to understand more of life and how individuals respond to it. For the sake of clarity, however, and despite the overlap, I will continue to discuss the role of the humanities under these two headings.

## Instrumental uses of the humanities

Instrumental uses can be divided into two groups: humanities subjects, particularly literature, can be seen as a source of case histories for medical students; and the humanities can teach students certain skills which may be of benefit to them in the clinical situation.

First, literature abounds with depictions of subjects relevant to medicine. The experience of depression is graphically portrayed in

*The Trick is to Keep Breathing* by Janice Galloway and in *The Bell Jar*, by Sylvia Plath; and the poems "Ambulances" and "The Building" by Philip Larkin describe what it is like to be a patient. Death and the experience of bereavement are frequent topics for writers such as Douglas Dunn in *Elegies* and CS Lewis in *A Grief Observed*. The advantage of studying works of literature rather than case studies of real patients is that the skill of the writer stimulates our imagination and arouses our sympathies, getting us involved with the characters and experiencing their trials with them.[12] Anne Scott has explored the idea of the development of the "moral imagination" in healthcare workers and has suggested that the study of literature may help to develop practitioners who are (in the words of Henry James) "finely aware and richly responsible".[13] By getting us involved with the characters, good literature can make students "finely aware" – a non-instrumental value in our context. But for literature to have an instrumental use we must take a further step to encourage students to consider how they would respond if they were to come across people with similar problems in professional practice and have responsibility for their care. This further step requires that students are directly challenged to consider their hypothetical responses to the fictional character or situation. This can be done in group work sessions and if the students" imaginations and feelings are already engaged, then the discussion will expose hidden prejudices and fears and allow discussion of the issues in a "safe" environment.

Second, how can literature and the humanities more generally teach useful skills which may be transferable to the medical context? Literature can teach about written communication but, more importantly for healthcare, drama demonstrates the nuances of communication between people, both verbal and non-verbal. Indeed, most communication skills courses now involve role play for the students with actors playing a part. Painting may also bring out the non-verbal ways in which feelings or attitudes can be expressed. The well-known painting "The Doctor" by Sir Luke Fildes illustrates eloquently the nature of the doctor–patient relationship. The doctor leans over his patient, a sick child, with a look of deep concentration in his face. The light in the picture focuses concern on these central characters while the parents stand, almost unnoticed, in the background.

History and philosophy may also train the students in useful skills. History can teach the importance of evidence and how it can be manipulated by individuals to give a fraudulent view of the truth. The medical world has become increasingly aware of fraud in medical research recently[14] and students may find it easier to perceive how evidence can be interpreted in different ways in a historical context. More specifically, the study of the history of medicine can remind students of the transient nature of much medical knowledge and of the importance of keeping up to date with developments. Philosophy (which is also important in the non-instrumental context) can teach students to order their thoughts, construct an argument and reach a logical conclusion. These skills are essential in diagnosis where the doctor must gather information to support a thesis and go through logical steps to reach a conclusion. I will illustrate this use of the humanities in the discussion of the philosophy module in the last part of this chapter.

## Non-instrumental value of the humanities

Turning now to the non-instrumental value of the humanities. I wish to argue that that value has three aspects: in education, and relatedly in personal development, and in providing the opportunity for students to step outside the pervasive ethos of the medical world and experience a kind of "counter-culture".

Turning first to the educational point, we can say that medicine is regarded as a "vocational" qualification at university in that it prepares students for a particular job at the end of their degree. We talk of students being "trained" to be doctors, rather than that they are being "educated" in medicine. It is important in this context to be aware of the distinctions between education and training and I will draw here on the work of the educational theorist RS Peters.[15] In a medical context, similar distinctions are drawn by Calman and Downie.[16] Briefly, to be educated is to have a broad perspective, as distinct from the narrow focus of training. Second, education is a process, not a single objective. As Peters says, "To be educated is not to have arrived; it is to travel with a different view."[17]

Peters' final point is that an educational process should be valuable as an end in itself and not just because it enables someone to do something else. When we speak of training the questions asked are: to be trained "in what" or trained to do what? But these questions do not fit the educational process.

These points were clearly in the minds of the GMC when they wrote *Tomorrow's Doctors*. Commenting on the deficiencies of current undergraduate medical education, they said that the current system resulted in a:

...regrettable tendency to underprovide those components of the course that are truly educational, that pertain to the proper function of a university and that are the hallmark of scholarship.[9]

Clearly, preparation for a career in medicine will involve some training as well as some educational activities and the GMC here pointed out that the latter have tended to be neglected. By allowing the study of literature, history or philosophy in the medical curriculum, we shall at the very least introduce breadth. But, more importantly, these subjects can challenge the students by introducing them to some of the great thinkers and will allow them to consider different ways of perceiving the world. This will encourage a critical and questioning attitude and help develop judgement.

Turning, secondly, to the value of the humanities in personal development, we can say that the educational process touches the student more deeply at a personal level than does the training process. Education is not just concerned with what someone can *do* but about what *kind of person* they become as a result of their education. Developing as a certain kind of person is important for the good doctor as medical practice is not just concerned with knowledge and skills but also with a humane and sympathetic approach to people. This is a quotation from the essay "On Liberty" by JS Mill.

> It really is of importance, not only what men do, but also what manner of men they are that do it. Among the works of men, which human life is rightly involved in perfecting and beautifying, the first of importance is man himself.[18]

It is here that a study of literature is best justified. As I have suggested, plays, poems and novels demand an emotional response from their readers and in doing so they will allow the students to discover their own hidden values and prejudices and to challenge them. This will encourage the kind of self-understanding ("fine awareness") which is essential for the development of mature human beings who are attuned and sympathetic to the perspectives and values of other people.

The final point about the non-instrumental value of the humanities is their role in providing the experience of a "counterculture" to medicine. Medical students often have the impression, and may be encouraged in it by their teachers, that they have an intellectual and moral superiority over other students. This is not helped by the fact that entrance requirements for medicine are amongst the highest in the university system or that medical students" university experience tends to be rather insular in that everyone follows the same course. The opportunity to take a humanities subject will allow medical students to meet teachers and students in other disciplines, will help reduce this isolation and may ultimately foster better relationships between doctors and the "outside world".

The GMC have now provided an opportunity for students to discover what the humanities have to offer within the structure of the curriculum. In their desire to increase the educational content of medical degrees, the GMC have suggested that arts and humanities subjects may be offered to students as part of their course in the form of special study modules.[19] These SSMs are to take up as much as one third of the total course and should be 4–5 week blocks set aside from the rest of the course to "allow the students to study in depth areas of particular interest to them". Examples of such modules and other structural ways in which the humanities can be made part of medical courses are mentioned below, but before doing so I would like to raise a point about the terminology of the "instrumental" and "non-instrumental".

Professor Raanan Gillon, in his editorial welcoming the appearance of the new journal *Medical Humanities*, offers a criticism of my argument that the humanities can have a non-instrumental value in medical education.[20] He does not dispute that the humanities can have a non-instrumental value; rather, his point is that if we are going to justify the inclusion of humanities in the medical curriculum it must be possible to show that in all cases they have an instrumental value for the curriculum, even if they are also valued for their own sake. He indicates that in the examples I give of the non-instrumental value of the humanities there is also an instrumental value.

In his chapter in this volume Robin Downie criticises the terminology of "instrumental" and "non-instrumental" (p.213). He accepts Gillon's point that if we are to justify the inclusion of the humanities in medical education we must be able to show what they contribute to the creation of the broadly educated doctor. His point is that it is a little misleading to see literature, for example, as "instrumental" in bringing about educatedness. Rather, the humanities are what he calls "component means" to the creation of the educated doctor. He gives the example of a painting and a paint brush. The paint brush is an instrumental means to the creation of the painting; it is a means in the sense that it is an important causal factor in the creation of the painting, but it is merely instrumental in the sense that when the painting is completed it has no continuing part in the painting. On the other hand, the colours of the painting are component means to the creation of the finished canvas and remain part of the organic whole. In a similar way, the humanities can be components in the creation of the educated doctor; they are there shaping the doctor's humane attitudes and furnishing a range of concepts and ways of seeing medicine which are complementary to the biomedical. This distinction between an instrumental means and a component means may enable me to meet Gillon's criticisms without losing my own point that the humanities can have justifications in different logical categories.

## Applications

Above I discussed justifications for the use of humanities in medical education and in this section I wish to consider the structural ways in which arts and humanities subjects can be included as part of a medical course. In doing this I will follow the conceptual model for medical humanities put forward by David Greaves in Chapter 1 but I will add another model to his list. Greaves considers two ways of seeing the application of arts and humanities in the medical educational context: the "additive" and the "integrative". The first refers to a situation where the arts subject is added on as a separate course within the curriculum. An example here would be some kinds of special study module. The integrative approach sees the medical humanities as giving the students a conceptual framework within which to understand all their medical studies: the biomedical *and* the vocational. I will add a third model to this list: the "complementary" approach. In this model, students are given an alternative point of view against which to pitch the medical model offered by their medical course. I will illustrate these three models with reference to some courses.

### The humanities as additive

Traditional medical courses have consisted of a great number of separate courses on different subjects. When I was in my fourth year at medical school we had 17 separate courses in the one year on subjects such as dermatology, ENT, and ophthalmology. Most medical curricula are now rationalising this situation by more carefully defining an essential "core" curriculum for medical students. The non-core subjects are now to be taught in the form of special study modules. There are no rules about what subject matter these should contain; rather, the main aim of the SSM should be educative and medical schools are encouraged by the GMC to make use of the "wider range of opportunities within their universities".[21] There is, therefore, the opportunity to offer courses in literature, history, foreign languages, philosophy and many other arts and humanities subjects.

When these courses are presented to students completely divorced from reference to their development as doctors, they could be described as "additive". In fact, very few SSMs can be described in this way as most have to be taught by medical or biomedical staff with a personal interest who are not professional teachers of literature, philosophy or history. The problem here is a practical one in that medical faculties are unwilling (as yet) to pay members of other faculties to contribute to the teaching, and teachers in humanities disciplines usually already have more than enough to do! One way of overcoming the time problem would be to allow medical students to take an entire course within another faculty and be examined on it as part of their degree. Money would have to flow between faculties but the students would get a high standard of teaching in their chosen subject rather than being instructed by enthusiastic amateurs.

Greaves is critical of this approach to the inclusion of the humanities, however, as the course is taken in complete isolation from the student's biomedical studies and there is no opportunity to affect the student's understanding of those studies. The problem is that the course becomes fragmentary and that science and art remain firmly fixed in their own separate boxes. This may prove so but I think that this view tends to underestimate the value of studying the humanities for a non-instrumental purpose. There is certainly a risk that if the relevance of the course to medical practice is not pointed out at each turn students will not make the connections, but some seeds may take root and grow[22] and, at the very least, the course will have some intrinsic value to the student as a university experience.

## The humanities as integrative

The integrative model sees the humanities as providing a context in which to understand medicine as a science, as an art and as a craft. This is clearly a more radical view of the part the humanities can play in medical education. Whereas the additive view sees the humanities as another course added on to what the students already do and as having a broadly educative value, the integrative view sees humanities as an integral and essential part of the course. This view implies that the medical humanities are part of the core curriculum.

Courses of this kind are beginning to emerge as developments of what are often called personal and professional development (PPD) modules within the core undergraduate curriculum.[23] These courses focus on the vocational and reflective aspects of the students" preparation to be doctors and involve ethics, communication, self-care, clinical reasoning and the understanding of how to integrate scientific knowledge about health and illness with personal and specific knowledge of a patient as a unique human being. Arts and humanities subjects are essential to such courses. Philosophy of medicine will help the students to understand the origins of medical knowledge and also the deficiencies of focusing entirely on scientific sources of evidence in medicine. Literature can provide case material for ethical debate and the experience of reading and discussing literary works will raise the students" awareness of the importance of interpretation in the medical encounter. Philosophy can provide a framework for ethics and also for more general logical analysis of medical problems. The aim of such a course is less to provide students with knowledge than to arm them with skills, methodologies, concepts, and self-awareness.

Another example of the integrative model in practice is the "Ethics in Medicine" SSM which is run as a compulsory course at the University of Aberdeen. This course includes the following amongst it core aims.

- To demonstrate that the resolution of ethical dilemmas in medical practice can be assisted by rational analysis, including the use of philosophical techniques.
- To introduce the concept that much learning, relevant to ethical dilemmas in medicine, can be gained from the study of various forms of the arts and humanities about why moral stances are taken by society and individuals.

There are as yet few examples in practice of the humanities as integrative, but it is likely to be a growth area in medical education in the next few years. These courses will require careful evaluation and there needs to be debate about this approach in the medical education journals.

## The humanities as complementary

In this model, the medical point of view is juxtaposed with an alternative view which is offered for the student's consideration. Most humanities SSMs are of this kind and aim to broaden the student's awareness of other conceptual approaches and other views and to extend their imaginations. Such courses depend on the students" ability to follow Forster's mantra "only connect".[24] John Berger's country doctor, Sassall, demonstrated his ability to make these imaginative connections in the book *A Fortunate Man*.[25] Sassall is described as "much influenced by the books of Conrad" and had been resolved as a child to become a sailor rather than a doctor. In this passage Berger described Sassall changing in his approach to medicine through making a connection with the experience of Conrad's Master Mariners.

> He began to realise that the way Conrad's Master Mariners came to terms with their imagination – denying it any expression but projecting it all on to the sea which they then faced as though it were simultaneously their personal justification and their personal enemy – was not suitable for a doctor in his position. He had done just that – using illness and medical dangers as they used the sea. He began to realise that he must face his imagination, even explore it. It must no longer always lead to the "unimaginable", as it had with the Master Mariners contemplating the possible fury of the elements – or, as in his case, to his contemplating only fights within the jaws of death itself. (The clichés are essential to the vision.) He began to realise that imagination had to be lived with on every level: his own imagination first – because otherwise this could distort his observation – and then the imagination of his patients.

In this complementary model, therefore, the humanities can be seen as holding up a mirror to the medical view of the world to encourage students to make comparisons, see similarities and be challenged by differences. One example of an SSM which attempted to do this is one on political philosophy which I was involved with at Glasgow University.[26] In this module students read the entire text of Plato's *Republic* and attended lectures in the philosophy department. The seminar discussions were based on themes dealt with in the *Republic* which had particular relevance to the students at this point in their course (second year). One theme was that of "The Family" and at this time the students were half way through their "Family Project" which involved them in a number of visits to a family and in reflection on the function of families in society. We were able to contrast Plato's radical view that the family had little importance in society with the view of our society (and also the current government) that the family was the backbone of society and provided its stability. The students were, therefore, led to challenge and question these prevailing views and commented in the evaluation that the module had taught them to question their views more.

Another example of the complementary model in action would be a module taught at the Royal Free and University College Medical School on "The Human Impact of the Genetic Revolution".[27] The aims of this module are to use literature, film, drama, and art to teach medical students:

- how the diagnosis of a genetic disorder impacts on the lives of patients and their families, and
- how to set this against the background of rapid and high-profile advances in the field of genetics and the historical record of the uses and abuses of knowledge of hereditary mechanisms.

The idea here is to make the students aware of the lay impact of medical advances in genetics by trying to get them to see these advances from the patient's point of view. In addition, the module uses history to challenge the view that scientific advance and new knowledge must always and necessarily be an unambiguously good thing.

The complementary model, then, can help stimulate the imaginations of students and get them to look at medical problems from another point of view. It is of value if the medical issue under consideration is linked in the curriculum to the time at which students take the module as this means that the issue is fresh in their minds. Unlike the integrative model, the complementary model does not pretend to provide a structure for understanding the rest of the course, but it may give students a methodology for analysing other problems and remind them of the importance of wider cultural awareness.

## Conclusion

These three structural models for the application of medical humanities within medical schools are all currently being used. The most common is the complementary, but the integrative is becoming more important. The first model, the additive, is the only one of the three which might be described as "non-instrumental" in its relationship to the development of students as doctors. All three models for the humanities will assist students in developing the wider toolkit of concepts and approaches to the practice of medicine that is now necessary for tackling the social determinants of health which are of increasing importance in developed societies in the 21st century.

## References and notes

1 Music therapy was granted professional status in 1999 through the Council for Professions Supplementary to Medicine (CPSM).
2 Wilkinson RG. *Unhealthy Societies.* London: Routledge, 1996: 4.
3 Social Exclusion Unit. *National Strategy for Neighbourhood Renewal: a framework for consultation.* London: Cabinet Office, 2000: 59.
4 Department of Health. *Saving Lives: our healthier nation.* London: HMSO, 1999.
5 Wilkinson[2], 1.
6 Matarasso, F. *Use or Ornament? The Social Impact of Participation in the Arts.* Stroud: Comedia, 1997: 14.
7 Downie RS. The role of literature in medical education. A commentary on the poem: Roswell, Hanger 84. *J Med Ethics* 1999; **25**: 529–31.
8 Broadie A. *The Scottish Enlightenment: an anthology.* Edinburgh: Canongate Classics, 1997: 757.
9 General Medical Council. *Tomorrow's Doctors: recommendations on undergraduate medical education.* London: GMC, 1993.
10 Gillon R. Imagination, literature, medical ethics and medical practice. *J Med Ethics* 1997; **23**: 3–4.
11 Evans M, Greaves D, Pickering N. Medicine, the arts and imagination (correspondence). *J Med Ethics* 1997; **23**: 254.
12 Downie R (ed.). *The Healing Arts.* Oxford: Oxford University Press, 1994: xvi.
13 Scott PA. Imagination in practice. *J Med Ethics* 1997; **23**: 45–50.
14 Lock S, Wells F (eds). *Fraud and Misconduct in Medical Research*, 2nd edn. London: BMJ Books, 1996.
15 Peters RS. *The Concept of Education.* London: Routledge and Kegan Paul, 1967; 31–7.
16 Calman KC, Downie RS. Education and training in medicine. *Med Educ* 1988; **22**: 488–91.
17 Peters[15], 8.

18  Mill JS. On liberty (1859). In Warnock M (ed.). *Utilitarianism*. Glasgow: Collins, 1962: 188.
19  GMC⁹, 9–10.
20  Gillon R. Welcome to medical humanities – and why (editorial). *J Med Ethics* 2000; **26**: 155–6.
21  GMC⁹, 9.
22  Macnaughton J. The humanities in medical education: context, outcomes and structures. *J Med Ethics: Med Humanities* 2000; **26**: 23–30.
23  The University of Sydney has such a course and the humanities are taking an ever greater role within it. The University of Durham is also developing a humanities-based PPD course for the new medical intake starting in October 2001.
24  Forster EM. *Howard's End*. Harmondsworth: Penguin Books, 1969.
25  Berger J. *A Fortunate Man*. New York: Vintage Books, 1967.
26  Downie R, Macnaughton J. Should medical students read Plato? *Med J Aust* 1999; **170**: 125–7.
27  The author is grateful to University College, London for sight of their course booklet for this course (1999).

# 13

# Medical humanities: means, ends, and evaluation

Robin Downie

Anyone who wishes to mount a course in the medical humanities for medical or nursing students, undergraduate or postgraduate, is going to be faced with a demand from deans or the like for the aims and evaluations of the courses. With a new subject this is not an unreasonable request. This chapter is therefore intended to make some suggestions about what can be said to sceptical deans, first about aims and second about evaluation. Third, I shall try to make a contribution to the debate on whether the medical humanities should be seen as means or ends in medical education.[1-3] I am concerned only with education and cannot comment on the use of the arts as therapy or in community work.

Three preliminary points must be made. First, for present purposes I shall use the terms "arts" and "humanities" interchangeably. Second, I shall stress that there are many different sorts of discipline which can be called "arts" or "humanities". Examples are archaeology, drama, the fine arts, history, languages, literature, medical history, music, philosophy, theology and so on. It will follow that there may be no one way of evaluating the contribution that such courses can make to the education of a healthcare professional. Equally, there will be no one dominant aim, unless it is something very wide, such as "to improve medical education". Some educational theorists would be happy with a few wide aims of this sort. They would then call "objectives" what I shall call "aims". I have no objection to this but will use only the term "aims" in this chapter. Third, enthusiasts for the medical humanities often say that the aim is to produce doctors who are more compassionate or who have empathy. But it is not at all clear that such aims can be achieved through a study of the humanities and certainly they cannot be evaluated. To be versed in the humanities is not the same as being humane, a point often illustrated by referring to Nazi officers. It might be more tellingly illustrated by inviting those of us who profess the humanities to consider ourselves and our colleagues and ask whether we are really more compassionate and humane than our medical colleagues. Some humility is required from those who claim from the safety of the study that doctors lack compassion and then seek to remedy this alleged defect by recommending a study of what we happen to be good at. I shall therefore suggest more concrete and realistic aims which those in the humanities might be in a position to help students and doctors achieve. In general terms, the hope would be to introduce students and doctors to a range of concepts and methods, other than narrowly scientific ones, which can assist with the understanding of human beings and their interactions and with doctor–patient communication. These aims can be placed into groups for convenience of discussion.

## Aims

### Group A: transferable skills

*To develop the ability to write clear English*

Medical English often has one or other or both of two faults. Either it is turgid and larded with professional terms or it is in bullet points. But when it comes to presenting a case to a wider audience then some attention to brevity and clarity and to what people might want to know is important. Perhaps such skills can be developed from courses on, say, journalism or writing.

*To develop sensitivity to nuances, ambiguities, and hidden meanings in ordinary conversation*

Some humanities, especially literature, involve concentration on language and a study of such disciplines will develop sensitivity to what patients may be saying. It is worth noting here that doctors and others who wish to promote the employment of the humanities in medical education are currently making the idea of "narrative" a central concept. Like the use of the term "evidence" by their scientifically-minded colleagues (see below) this wide use of "narrative" obscures as much as it illuminates. In the brief time a doctor spends with a patient in a consultation the patient might relate a short anecdote, but there is not likely to be much time for anything that would justify the grand term "narrative", unless perhaps in psychotherapy. Doctors who wish to learn from the humanities might do well to become aware of the range of conceptual tools which are available – from hermeneutics, rhetoric, linguistics, and so on – rather than march behind generalised slogans such as "the patient's narrative". There are many other concepts which might more precisely direct the doctor's attention to the nature and implications of the language used by the patient.[4]

*To develop the ability to analyse arguments, justify clinical decisions and present cases clearly to a lay public*

This aspect of the humanities is of course very familiar through the efforts of those who have been involved in the development of medical ethics over several decades. Indeed, the new medical humanities movement stands in an uneasy relationship with the older medical ethics movement. Is ethics to be taught separately from the humanities or is ethics one aspect of humanities teaching? There are practical and organisational questions here which medical faculties need to address. But the point in this context is that philosophy is undoubtedly a humanity and it is philosophers who can offer guidance in the analysis of arguments.

*To develop the ability to assess different sorts of evidence*

It cannot be overemphasised at the moment that the evidence from randomised clinical trials is only one sort of evidence relevant to clinical judgement. A historian, say, or a detective will look for a different sort of evidence – one related to the specific incident or event – and their sort of evidence may be logically closer to the kind which influences a clinician, who is dealing with this particular patient, than the evidence of trials, which is generalised. In general, science works with one sort of evidence – mainly inductive – but the humanities can introduce doctors to other sorts which are equally relevant to the practice of medicine.[5]

*To develop the ability to see connections between apparently disparate situations*

EM Forster's novel *Howard's End* states its overriding theme before the book starts: "Only connect". And the story illustrates the tragic consequences when the characters fail to do this.[6]

## Group B: the humanistic perspective

*To enable students to develop broad perspectives on human beings and society, which place medical practice into a wider context or put it into a social framework*

There are many different ways of seeing human beings of which the scientific is only one and there are many different ways of seeing society of which a western liberal way is only one. For example, I was involved in teaching a special study module (SSM) on Plato's *Republic*.[7] It so happened that the medical students had just finished their "Family Project", a project which presupposed the importance of the family unit. They were then faced with Plato's arguments against the family. It was salutary for them to appreciate that not everyone thinks that the family and family values are good and to be obliged to make explicit and defend the values which their project was presupposing.

The development of broad perspectives may be especially important in medicine because, like the military and the police, medicine has its own ethos and bonding is encouraged. There is therefore a tendency to develop narrow perspectives and to close ranks. In the present age this can be undesirable.

### To develop moral sensitivity

The teaching of medical ethics has tended to fall into the hands of philosophers. But philosophers are interested in general principles and theories which have a limited appeal to medical students because of their abstract and generalised nature. On the other hand, literature or film can make a much more powerful impact on moral awareness because of its immediacy. Like medicine itself literature deals with the details of cases. Indeed, there is a danger that philosophy actually blunts moral awareness because students become caught up with terms such as "deontology" or "patient autonomy" or with the technicalities of moral argument which blind them to the reality of the situations they will be dealing with. I have discussed this elsewhere.[8]

## Group C: coping with the particular situation

*To develop the ability to understand and to cope with particular situations where rules and guidelines do not exactly apply*

In this context it is helpful to refer to Plato's discussion in Book X of the *Republic* of an "ancient quarrel" between philosophers on the one hand and poets and dramatists on the other.[9] The quarrel concerns the qualifications of each to make recommendations about the nature of the good life. Plato has no doubt that poets and dramatists are trying to do the same sort of thing as the philosophers (otherwise there would be no quarrel) but he holds that they lack proper understanding for the job. Plato's view is that real understanding comes from having insight into the blueprints, the timeless patterns, which make things as they are. In our day the task of discovering such patterns has been taken up by scientists and of course doctors are keen to follow the lead of scientists.

Now Plato's arguments against the humanities as a source of knowledge or understanding are limited because they depend on his assumption that the arts and humanities are essentially imitative, an assumption which would not nowadays be accepted. But even those who do not make that assumption may agree with Plato that the arts are not a source of real understanding. In terms of this point of view the arts are to be seen as decorative or entertaining or expressive of emotion. But this position can be challenged. It can be maintained that the arts and humanities can provide a distinctive sort of understanding, an understanding of the particular situation, and the qualitative distinctions involved. Let us examine this sort of understanding.

Literature, drama, and film are concerned above all with qualitative distinctions. There is no one measure or scale in terms of which the interaction of the characters can be measured. One event or action is not just a different quantity of another; rather, novels, plays, and films are concerned with the qualitative richness of human interaction and the possibilities for tragedy involved. Moreover, literature shows us that in order to understand any particular action or character it is necessary to see the interrelatedness of them all. This kind of understanding is quite different from the understanding generated by science, which enables us to understand by demonstrating the patterns or laws which cover individual events or changes. Social science tries to do the same, perhaps less certainly, for human actions. But such understanding is achieved only if we abstract from the complexity of human motivation and interaction. For example, "rational economic man" is not any man of flesh and blood but an abstraction. But he is an explanatory concept in economics, just as "the role of the patient" and its associated behaviours is thought to be explanatory in medical sociology. But although this may help to explain the behaviour of Hamish MacTavish who has just been admitted to hospital it may also mislead since it is abstracted from the complex motivation and interrelatedness of this specific individual. It is in literature or drama or film that we find this distinctive sort of understanding pre-eminently illustrated. It is a genuine kind of understanding, but quite distinct from that provided by science or social science. Through imaginative identification with the characters in a story or play we can develop the capacity for insights into the human condition with which medicine is concerned.

## Group D: self-awareness

*To develop self-awareness, including awareness of one's own emotions*

One criticism of doctors is that they are not always aware of how they are coming across to patients; and one problem of some doctors is emotional burn-out, which is not only self-destructive but also has a bad effect on patients. What we call a person's inner life is the inside story of his own history, the way living in the world feels to him. This kind of experience is usually only vaguely known, because most of its components are nameless, and it is hard to form an idea of anything which has no name. This easily leads to the conclusion that feeling is entirely formless, that it has causes which may be determined, and effects which must be dealt with (sometimes by drugs) but that it itself is irrational, a disturbance of the organism with no structure of its own. Yet subjective experience has a structure which can be reflected on and symbolically expressed. It cannot be expressed through the discursive – everyday or scientific – use of language but it can be known through the arts.

Works of art are expressive forms and what they express is the nature of human feeling. The arts make our inner subjective life visible, audible or in some other way perceivable, through symbolic form.[10] What is artistically good is what articulates and presents feeling to our understanding. Note that while an artist expresses feeling it is not as a baby might. The artist objectifies subjective life. What the artist expresses is not his own feelings but what he knows about feeling. A work of art expresses a conception of life, emotion, and inward reality. That is why the arts can help to create the self-understanding which is important for any doctor dealing with vulnerable human beings. As JS Mill puts it: "It really is of importance, not only what men do, but also what manner of men they are that do it".[11]

## Group E: joint investigation

*To experience the process of joint investigation*

All the aims so far discussed have been in terms of the outcomes of studying the humanities. But it is arguable that for some subjects the outcomes in terms of new knowledge or skills are less important than the process by which these outcomes are approached. In the humanities, or some of them, it is possible for the student to challenge the point of view of the teacher to an extent that would not be possible in a subject such as biochemistry. This is not the same as learning to work in a team (which is important but is learned elsewhere). The study of the humanities can involve a joint exploration in which students can put forward points of view which can then be modified in the light of what their peers say. The result might be that all members of the study group, including the teacher or facilitator, reach a more considered understanding than they had before. The point here is the nature of what is learned in the process of discussion rather than the outcome. Process-led approaches to higher education have been proposed by Stenhouse[12] and more recently by Laurillard.[13]

# Evaluation

Undergraduate and postgraduate students can of course evaluate a course in familiar ways, by means of questionnaires and so on. The main problem, however, is the one with which the educator is faced. Has the course been educationally worthwhile and for what reasons? How can this kind of evaluation proceed?

In one sense there is no difficulty about evaluating a medical humanities course. It can be assessed by examination or essay or other project. This has happened in arts faculties for centuries and there is a great deal of experience in arts faculties of this sort of evaluation. The difficulty in a medical context is really that of the standard which can be expected. SSMs usually last about five weeks and involve intensive study of one subject. What kind of standard is it reasonable to expect, granted that a medical student may have no background in the subject? There is the connected problem of who the teachers should be. It is unlikely that doctors will undertake teaching in linguistics, say, or archaeology but they may well teach literature (which is an instant-expert subject!).

Of course here the educational theorists may object that the whole concept of "teaching" is outmoded, or "didactic" (a damning term in educational circles). They might go on to suggest that the problem of who the teachers should be can be avoided if students are set problems and learn for themselves by attempting to answer them, perhaps with a "facilitator". But the facilitator must still set the tasks and evaluate the outcomes, so the question remains of what the educational background of this person should be. The best solution to all this would be for medical students to be given the opportunity to sit in on an arts faculty subject for a session and be taught by arts faculty staff and evaluated along with other arts faculty students. But for time-tabling and other reasons this will rarely be possible. In most cases what is likely to happen is that interested medical staff will mount SSMs in literature or the like and the students will be evaluated by medical staff. There is a risk, of course, that such courses run by medical facilitators will be seen by humanities staff as substandard both in academic content and in the level attained by the students; indeed, both may be the case. But the courses may still be worth doing.

Even supposing we have secured agreement at this first level of evaluation we must face a harder problem. Deans will need to be shown what a study of the humanities can do for the professional life of doctors. How can you become a better doctor by a study of the humanities? To ask this question is to ask how a skill or knowledge can be transferred from its base in a humanities subject to a medical context. The answer will depend on the particular subject we are concerned with. Some skills may transfer very easily. For example, a class in writing or in journalism may succeed in developing the skill to describe a case or write an information sheet for patients which is clear and comprehensible. Clear writing is a skill which can transfer because it is the same skill in any context and can have the same criteria for evaluation. Equally, it might be possible in a philosophy module to develop the skill to analyse an argument and be able to state its strong or weak points. This is an obviously transferable skill which can be evaluated in a manner appropriate for a medical context. In other words, most of the aims mentioned in Group A can be shown to transfer to the medical context, where their relevance is clear, and they can be evaluated in a medical context.

Other skills are not so obviously transferable and the problem of evaluation for a medical curriculum is therefore harder. For example, how can we evaluate what the study of a poem might do for the training of a doctor? Let us begin with how it might be evaluated in an arts faculty context. The poem would be read and perhaps some account might be given of the background, the historical period and other works by the poet. Discussion of the poem would concentrate on its ambiguities of meaning, its imagery, its rhythm and rhyme scheme, and how they support the meaning of the poem. Students might then be asked to write an essay on the poem and a good essay might suggest that it was open to three interpretations but that the prevailing imagery supported one of the interpretations. There is no inherent problem about evaluating an essay of this sort. Indeed, another essay taking a different line might be evaluated just as highly provided its argument was coherent and supported by good textual and background evidence. Can skills of this kind transfer to a medical context and can they be shown to do so? Medical students might need some help in making the transfer. Indeed, many doctors are highly cultured in the sense that they appreciate music, read poetry and novels and so on. But they do not see the relevance of this to the practice of medicine. Some time might therefore be profitably spent in showing a student that the ambiguities we can detect in a poem might also be found in the words of patients. The ability to make these links can perhaps be evaluated. "Only connect"!

## Ends and means

It is clear that some medical humanities can be evaluated easily in terms of their contribution to medical education – those especially in Group A. Other groups might be harder to evaluate, but it seems intuitively plausible that they would contribute to medical education and could therefore be seen as conducive to the creation of a good doctor. At this point a humanist might object that the humanities are worthwhile for their own sake. The humanist could cite Aristotle who develops a distinction between activities which are justified by their instrumentality in bringing about further ends, and the highest good, a good-in-itself, an intrinsic good or a "final end".[14] One criterion for belonging to that category is that the activity in question must be totally useless! Aristotle's argument is that if an activity is useful its justification is in terms of what it produces, so it cannot be good-in-itself. It follows that the highest good must be good in and for itself and not for its usefulness. Now Aristotle places "contemplation" (which means something like pure philosophy) in that category (although not ethics, which is a guide to a good life). Many people might want to place the arts in the same category.

In the light of this distinction between an instrumental good – something good as a means – and an intrinsic good – something good as an end, what can we say about the place of the humanities in medical education? I have so far categorised the aims of humanities teaching and their evaluation in terms of an apparent instrumentality. Does that mean that the literature, drama and so on in these courses are not worthwhile for their own sake?

In her contribution to the first number of *Medical Humanities* Dr Jane Macnaughton distinguishes between the instrumental uses of the humanities in medical education (such as those mentioned in my Group A) and their non-instrumental aspects.[2] She mentions three of what she considers the non-instrumental values: broadening educational horizons, for example by introducing students to alternative ways of seeing the world (my Group B); assisting in the personal development of students and doctors (my Group D); and the introduction of a "counterculture" (my Group B). I might also add the ability to understand human beings and their interactions in an irreducibly qualitative way, an ability, I allege, which can be developed by appreciation of the arts (my Group C). The points Dr Macnaughton is making are that certain humanities studies are worthwhile for their own sake but should be included in medical education despite the fact, or even because of the fact, that they are non-instrumental.

Now in the *Journal of Medical Ethics* Professor Gillon has written a very generous editorial welcoming the appearance of *Medical Humanities*.[3] In this he takes Dr Macnaughton to task over her instrumental/non-instrumental distinction. He is not denying the intrinsic value of the arts and humanities; indeed, he is asserting that they have such an intrinsic value. He is making two points: that the humanities should not be included in medical education unless they have an instrumental value, but that *in addition* to their intrinsic value the humanities do in fact have an instrumental value for medical education. And he goes on to claim that Dr Macnaughton's three examples of the non-instrumental values of the arts for doctors are in fact "surely open to interpretation as being highly 'instrumentally' valuable (quite apart from their intrinsic value) in the simple sense of being likely to produce better doctors and therefore appropriately introduced in medical education for that purpose". He then goes on to show how this is the case in her three types of example (and I have no doubt that he would say the same over my Group C cases of a special type of understanding).

Professor Gillon's argument seems plausible but only if we grant him two assumptions: that we can stretch the meaning of "instrumental" until it is really very thin; and that something can be at one and the same time instrumentally good and an intrinsic good or "final end". If we take his first assumption we can see what I am calling the "thinness" of his use of the concept of instrumentality when he says that something is "instrumental" if it conduces to human flourishing or to a better understanding of the outside world or to personal development. This application of "instrumental" is far removed from baseline applications of the concept, as when we say that a hack-saw was instrumental in the prisoner's escape or that the headmaster was instrumental in influencing the pupil's choice of career. The baseline use of "instrumental" has two features: it implies that there is a causal connection between the instrument and what its use leads to, and it implies that the instrument has no place in the end brought about by its use. Neither of these conditions holds when we say, for example, that the appreciation of the arts conduces to human development. The term "conduces" does not here indicate a causal connection, for a causal connection would imply that the appreciation of the arts was one thing and human development something different. The point is, however, that an appreciation of the arts is a necessary component part of the final end state of human development or of educatedness. Hence, the language of instrumentality is misleading because of its associations with causality. The second assumption is also debatable – that something can be causally instrumental and also a final end. I do not want to press this, however, partly because I do not wish to engage in a discussion over the interpretation of Aristotle but mainly because I believe the entire controversy is misconceived; it seems real only because of the terminology in which it is stated. In short, I wish to maintain that the distinction between an instrumental means and an intrinsic or final end is misleading.

Consider the following example, that of the creation of a painting. In painting a picture the artist will use assorted instrumental means, such as paint brushes, an easel and, say, a model. These are instruments whose justification lies in the final end or product – the painting. They are causally or productively connected with the painting and when it is completed they have no further part to play (unless, of course, the painting is being entered for the Turner Prize!). As instrumental means they are only contingently connected with the painting and are removed leaving no trace when it is finished. Is Professor Gillon saying that Dr Macnaughton's examples are instrumental in that sense? That literature and so on are only causally or contingently or extrinsically connected with producing a flourishing or educated human being and when they have done their work they will be removed like the easel, etc.? Obviously not! But that is the implication of using the terminology of instrumentality.

What then should be said? Let us return to the example of the painting. The paint brushes, easel, model, etc. are instrumental means to the painting and have no part to play when it is completed. But the canvas, paint and the shapes it creates are also means to the creation of the painting. The difference is that they do have a necessary part in the finished product. We can therefore call them component (as distinct from instrumental) means to the painting. In Aristotle's terminology, the paint brushes, etc. are efficient causes of the painting whereas the canvas, paint, and shapes are the material and formal causes of the painting, which itself is the final cause, the ultimate aim of the whole process.[15]

If we apply these distinctions to the question of the relationship between the humanities, the educated person, and the good doctor it might be possible to take the following line. We can say that the enjoyment and practice of the humanities are activities worthwhile for their own sake and that they are means to creating an educated, developed, flourishing human life. But they are not instrumental in that process; they are essential components of such a life. To put it another way, we can say that part of what it means to be an educated developed human being is to be able to enjoy at least some humanities for their own sake. Of course, that is only part of what it means; there are other essential components in the educated life, such as some appreciation of science, some interest in current affairs, some general curiosity, and so on. For the developed or flourishing life other aspects would also be needed, such as friends.

It is a separate question (often overlooked by those teaching the humanities) whether it is necessary for a good doctor to be an educated, developed human being. Perhaps doctors should simply be highly trained with highly specialised skills. Perhaps the ability to look before and after just gets in the way and distracts from the technical business of medicine. Certainly this would be true of some scientists, who have devoted their entire lives to pursuing some scientific or mathematical goal at the cost of every other side to their nature. This is one kind of good life from which we all benefit. Can the same be true of some doctors? Perhaps of some doctors, but to the extent that doctors must deal with patients, with other human beings, they differ from scientists or mathematicians. This does not mean that they must be overflowing with compassion or empathy, because these are inward-looking concepts. An analogy with playing an instrument might help. The good musician, giving a moving performance, is not brimming with emotion – he would lose the place if he were! His feelings are, as it were, in his fingers. So with the doctor; his gaze should be outward, away from himself. The doctor needs to be aware of what is on the whole likely to be good for this particular patient and requires sensitivity to the patient's wishes, consent or refusal and so on. In other words, the doctor needs to be able to make considered judgements, and a developed sense of judgement has a humanistic element as a component means.[5]

# References and notes

1   Evans M, Greaves D, Pickering N. Medicine, the arts and imagination (correspondence). *J Med Ethics* 1997: **23**; 254.
2   Macnaughton J. The humanities in medical education: context, outcomes and structures. *J Med Ethics: Med Humanities* 2000; **26**:23–30.
3   Gillon R. Welcome to medical humanities – and why (editorial). *J Med Ethics* 2000; **26**; 155–6.
4   Culler J. *Literary Theory*. Oxford: Oxford University Press, 1997.
5   Downie R, Macnaughton J. *Clinical Judgement: evidence in practice*. Oxford: Oxford University Press, 2000.
6   Forster EM. *Howard's End*. Harmondsworth: Penguin Books, 1969.
7   Downie R, Macnaughton J. Should medical students read Plato? *Med J Aust* 1999; **170**: 125–7.
8   Downie R. The role of literature in medical education. *J Med Ethics* 1999; **25**: 529–31.
9   Plato. *Republic*. London: Sphere Books, 1970: Book X.
10  Langer SK. *Feeling and Form*. London: Routledge and Kegan Paul, 1953.
11  Mill JS. On liberty (1859). In: Warnock M (ed.). *Utilitarianism*. Glasgow: Collins, 1962: 188.
12  Stenhouse L. *An Introduction to Curriculum Research and Development*. London: Heinemann, 1975.
13  Laurillard D. *Rethinking Teaching*. London: Routledge, 1993.
14  Aristotle. *Nicomachean Ethics*. New York: Random House, 1941: 1097a-b.
15  Aristotle. *Physics*. New York: Random House, 1941: Book II, Chapter 3.

# Section 4
# Understanding Medical Knowledge

*Introduction*                                                     219

14  Validating the facts of experience in medicine                 223

15  The humanities' role in improving health and
    clinical care                                                  236

16  Philosophy and the medical humanities                          250

# Introduction

This last section considers one of the more theoretical ideas at stake in this book – namely that engagement with the humanities affects not just how medicine might be practised, but also how its nature might be understood. Is medicine an essentially scientific endeavour, practised in an interpersonal context, which must be made "user friendly" by taking account of the sensitivities of patient and practitioner alike? Or is medicine an essentially humanistic endeavour, whose goals concern experiential aspects of human existence; an endeavour that is practised in a scientific context that must be made as systematic and rigorous as possible, provided that the individuality of patients is attended to first and foremost?

Whilst the primary purpose of this book is to stimulate and encourage thinking about how the humanities can be incorporated into a richer *practice*, there is a role for theoretical considerations as well. For beyond an initial and probably widely agreed sensitising of medicine's processes, our view of the scope and prospects for further "humanising" medical practice will reflect what we take to be the nature of medicine itself. Thus the choice between an essentially scientific and an essentially humanistic conception of medicine has important implications for how far, and in what ways, we will think medical practice ought to embody the insights of the humanities. For these reasons, we regard it as important to include this more theoretical section.

At stake is the question of how medical knowledge ought to be conceived and understood. The first contribution to this section, by physician John Saunders, tackles this question head on from within a medical perspective, as we shall see. It involves an explicitly philosophical undertaking; the second contribution is a personal reflection upon the relation between science, the humanities, and the healthcare of populations and individuals from Richard Edwards, recently retired Director of Research and Development for health and social care in Wales. The final chapter reflects on the particular engagement of the humanities with medicine and the contribution of this dialogue, from the viewpoint of a philosopher, Martyn Evans.

To begin with the first of these contributions, it is evident that medicine unites anecdotal interest in individual persons with mathematical interest in the complexity of molecular biology. Clinical medicine and medical education need both cognitive (rational) and affective (emotional) threads which do not simply align with the objective and the subjective. Saunders explores how these two threads are united in *personal knowing*, an important though difficult notion which itself summons a philosophical understanding of the unity of our culture.

Personal participation and imagination are essentially involved in science as well as in humanities; meanings which are created in science are, in this respect, no more privileged than meanings created in humanities; imagination and personal participation are central to both. For the philosopher of science Michael Polanyi, the processes of knowing are exhibited first in the choice of a problem and thereafter all the way to verification of discovery. For Saunders, following Polanyi, the real methods of science are not detachment but commitment and involvement. Practical knowledge, irreducibly involved in science, makes this evident (knowing how to ride a bicycle is fundamentally different from (perhaps incompatible with) specifying how to do it) as, for instance, in instructing someone else. Something similar, explains Saunders, is true for all knowledge, both in the sciences and in the humanities. We know a whole *through* its parts, which we absorb and adopt, rather than by focusing our attention upon each of them. Seen like this, the humanities are not *added* to science but both are part of a common culture. In both contexts of knowledge, we understand the world from our individual points of view, claiming originality, exercising personal judgement and responsibility.

The need for a closer union between medicine and the humanities, and its implications, are considered by Richard Edwards. Despite, indeed perhaps because of, the advances in biomedical science, popular consumer expectations of medicine remain largely unsatisfied in the face of high spending on healthcare. The narrative dimensions of health and illness elude the reductionist scientific grounding of evidence-based medicine, tempting people to seek help from "alternative" therapies and, to an extent, to mistrust scientific medical care. People seek from such alternative therapies a richer professional contact than is routinely available within scientific medicine. The gap between the "organism" and the whole patient might still be bridged, however, if an understanding of the humanities were integrated within our scientific conception of organised healthcare.

The humanities constitute forms of "language" for the communication of emotion and experience, and these can and should be incorporated into our conception of such healthcare delivery. In particular, there should be greater emphasis on the "stories" by which patients understand themselves and their health needs; such narrative can and should reflect the capabilities of science, conveying them more effectively. Moreover stories give people self-expression. Literature can disclose and explore the context and unfolding activities of the sciences. Literature moreover provides us with a wealth of narrative regarding the variety of experiences of health and illness, medical care and the perspectives of patient and doctor alike. Significantly it reveals the uncomfortable links sometimes found between pathology and creativity.

The humanities can also be regarded together as a whole; as such they offer records of collective experience and resources for dealing with life's challenges. Such challenges do not take merely economic forms, nor are they necessarily amenable to economic solutions; creative responses to them involve the fulfilment of a wider range of personal aspirations. Whether or not directly expressing concerns with health and illness, the opportunities which the humanities offer for creative engagement make a valuable contribution to the promotion of individual and collective health.

If one discipline claims more than any other to be concerned with thinking about how we *ought to think* about practices such as medicine, that discipline is philosophy. Martyn Evans considers how philosophy as a discipline is regarded or understood and reviews a number of philosophical questions concerning the nature of medicine itself, including the question of whether, and how, the humanities belong at the core of medical knowledge. Such questions are inherently philosophical. They may be considered instrumentally, that is, for the sake of practical benefits which might follow from clarifying them, or intrinsically, that is, for the sake of the enriched sense of wonderment which might follow from a consideration of the nature of "the human", as medicine confronts it. Considerations of this type involve our enquiring both into the nature of the world as we experience it and into *how* we can know about it and, in our different ways, value it. In such terms, medicine and philosophy share a role in our attempts to understand ourselves as both physical and rational, experiential beings – embodied selves.

Philosophy's modern engagement with medicine began with an interest in "medical ethics". It was soon realised that such questions inevitably lead to considering medicine's nature, goals, and characteristic knowledge base and to our attempting to conceptualise the human body and indeed "the human" more generally. Recently, discussion of values has widened beyond ethics, using philosophy as a tool, to consider human values in health and medicine and the component aesthetic, political, social, intellectual and gustatory values, among others. Philosophy's core practices of critical reflection provide a consistent rigour in the quest to understand these diverse values in modern clinical medicine – marking philosophy's place among the "medical humanities" as a central one.

# 14

# Validating the facts of experience in medicine

John Saunders

> Medicine spans the two ends of the art-science spectrum. One
> foot is planted in the physical world, electronic impulses and
> muck of the human body; the other is planted in the subjective,
> experiential world of consciousness and conduct.[1]

It is this dual nature of medicine that constitutes its attraction to so
many of its practitioners and students. The anecdotal human
interest on the one hand contrasts with the mathematical
complexities of the new genetics and molecular biology; the
opportunity to master skills contrasts with the chemical or
engineering principles which underlie them and make them
possible and effective.

## Doctors and the new technologies

New knowledge has given rise to new problems for human beings
and a growth industry in bioethics. New technologies create
possibilities of new experiences for people: artificial organs and
limbs, new psychological states, survival with new disabilities. New
skills arise in response to engineering advances: laparoscopic
surgery, endoscopic diagnostic techniques and treatments. The
doctor as healer, as a humane rounded fellow creature, needs to
know more and soon seems to change into a technician. Not all
technologies are successful; not all new drugs are effective; the
indications for this and that become more and more refined. The
costs rise and the cry goes out for evidence: more evidence, better
evidence. We now live in an age of "evidence-based medicine".
Feeding this desire for evidence are new journals, broadsheets,
meetings, guidelines, and rising medicolegal threats. It would

hardly be surprising if doctors were less reflective, more concentrated on the need to absorb the latest available information in the field, less open to insights from the humanities, more concerned with measurement, less empathic to the experiences which the new advances can produce.

Is this true? Of course, we don't know. School leavers entering our medical schools remain among the most talented of our young people, often gifted in subjects far beyond those of biology and mathematics. Yet the crowded medical curriculum, both before and after graduation, has given rise to concerns that the volume of information that needs to be absorbed deadens the creative spirit, dulls the enthusiasm, and reorientates priorities towards the measurable and the technical. And despite much rhetoric about "holistic" medicine, it is undeniable that more and more patients are treated by committee, as one specialist refers to another. Even the simplest problem in another specialist's patch seems to generate another referral. That certainly makes it easy to lose the personal: "I'm only looking after the patient's legs". Given medicine's nature, is it possible to move away from an obsession with evidence, construed as numbers, from Thomas Gradgrind's philosophy of knowledge as facts?

> "Now, what I want is, Facts. Teach these boys and girls nothing but Facts. Facts alone are wanted in life. Plant nothing else, and root out everything else. You can only form the minds of reasoning animals upon Facts: nothing else will ever be of any service to them... Stick to Facts, sir!"... Thomas Gradgrind. With a rule and a pair of scales, and the multiplication table always in his pocket, sir, ready to weigh and measure any parcel of human nature, and tell you exactly what it comes to... he seemed a kind of cannon loaded to the muzzle with facts, and prepared to blow them clean out of the regions of childhood at one discharge. He seemed a galvanising apparatus, too, charged with a grim mechanical substitute for the tender young imaginations that were to be stormed away.[2]

Is it possible to move away from Gradgrind's dour philosophy, from a conception of medical knowledge as ticking boxes in some lifelong multiple choice exam, to one of wisdom?

Williams[3] describes this in different terms, from the religious believer's perspective:

Medicine and the life of faith have something to say to each other and to society around them...not every anguish, not every crisis, is a problem that can be solved by throwing information at it. Our humanity seems to cope with its problems more by listening, intuition, relationship, than by detached skills and the acquiring of facts alone...some commitments just aren't possible without a deeper commitment to what the human community is like, what kind of beings human beings are.

If this is the case, he goes on, the community of faith is concerned with medicine as "a set of conversational and relational skills, rooted in but not confined by knowledge of the material organism" and also with "the national guaranteeing of healthcare, as a sign of society's willingness to confront weakness and mortality without fear". In an era of stunning advances in material knowledge, humanity is misunderstood.

... the humanity in view is a humanity rather different from what a lot of our late modernity seem to take for granted – hasty, anxious, obsessed with measurable successes, deeply embarrassed by failure and death... It isn't easy to sustain the humane vision of medicine (or anything else) when the rules of our humanity are apparently being rewritten to suit the imperatives of management and profit.

## Acquiring a "medical" education

It might be suggested, then, that courses in medicine need two threads or aspects: the cognitive and the affective,[4] which are not at all the same as the objective and the subjective. In their cognitive aspect, medical courses should aim to challenge dogmatism, to broaden perspectives and to oppose the myth of a non-scientific free-for-all.[5] In its affective aspect, such courses should cultivate individual, social, and cultural understanding, to encourage an empathic emotional awareness. This duality is essential to proper doctoring. Yet this may not be enough. An education in the arts and an appreciation of another sphere of human endeavour do not guarantee a reverence for human beings or an appreciation of our science as an essentially human and personal activity. It has been said that "nothing in the next door world of Dachau impinged on the great winter cycles of Beethoven chamber music played in Munich. No canvases came off the museum walls as the butchers strolled reverently past, guide book in hand".[6]

Do liberal attitudes make individuals more cultured or vice versa? And if we believe these two *are* related, how do these affective qualities relate to the cognitive content of our courses? If we can understand our knowing as personal knowing, as a commitment we affirm to an external reality, may this enable us to bridge the two cultures described by CP Snow,[7] to unite medicine with the humanities and not to separate it from them? If we are to affirm the place of the humanities in medicine, we also need a philosophical understanding of the unity of our culture.

## Scientific medicine

"Modern medicine in industrialised countries is scientific medicine. The claim, tacitly made by American and European doctors and tacitly relied on by their patients, is that their palliatives and procedures have been shown by science to be effective. Medical practice depends on generalisations that can be reliably applied and scientifically demonstrated. Without understanding people as objects in this way, there can be no such thing as medical science."[8]

But there is a problem with evidence, however desirable it may be: problems of absolute versus relative differences, of publication bias, of meta-analysis, subgroup analysis, equivalence testing, problems of why we measure one thing rather than another and how we select the subjects we study in the first place. For example, to decide to express data as showing a relative difference (x cures twice as many as something else) rather than an absolute difference (x cures 1% rather than 0.5%) is not an issue that the computer can solve for you. Or again, positive results favouring a new treatment are more likely to be published than negative ones. Meta-analysis is a way of combining results from small studies, a way to put all available information together. Unfortunately, the contributory studies to the analysis may have had a variety of different characteristics. Putting them together may look good statistically but can resemble adding apples and pears. In the case of subgroup analysis, clinical trial results are reanalysed to see if a significant finding can be discovered for a particular subgroup – identified by age, gender, other pathologies, severity of the pathology under test or indeed anything. The ISIS-2 trial, involving

17 187 patients, showed the value of streptokinase in patients with acute myocardial infarction. In a subgroup whose astrological birth sign was Gemini or Libra, the death rate was higher on the placebo. All the benefit from the streptokinase in the trial was gained by those patients with other birth signs. Presumably this is nonsense. Hampton discusses this at length with other examples in his 1997 Fitzpatrick Lecture.[9]

None of these problems is soluble by a mechanistic approach according to the canons of objectivism. In addition, uncertainty increases when several therapeutic agents or techniques are combined into a clinical management strategy.[10] Two agents or techniques can be assessed in two different sequences, yet five agents give 120 sequence options. No trial can explore the latter and anyway a new treatment will have arrived by the time it does. By the canons of objectivism, nobody knows, or could know, how to treat rheumatoid arthritis or diabetes. But if this exemplifies the difficulty of even establishing generalisations, how much harder is it to validate the facts of our experience in treating individual patients? Here perhaps is the most fundamental flaw in the doctrines of evidence-based practice. Charlton wrote:

> The basic error of evidence based medicine is quite simple. It is that epidemiological data do *not* provide the information necessary to treat individual patients. The error is intractable and intrinsic to the methodological nature of epidemiology, and no amount of statistical jiggery-pokery with huge data sets can make any difference.[11]

Consider this example in a medical newspaper.[12] A Norfolk physician pointed out that the largest trial of antihypertensive therapy studied 17 000 patients with mild hypertension for over 90 000 patient-years of accumulated treatment. There was no benefit in lives saved and 850 patient-years of treatment were needed to prevent one stroke. Expressed differently, of 25 people on treatment for 35 years, one will benefit. Thus, he calculated, 24 people will take 38 325 pills each, a total of 919 800 pills or, laid end to end, three miles of tablets of no proven benefit. As he observed, most of us measure our gin consumption in units per week rather than swimming pools per lifetime. Nevertheless, this example does suggest a different perspective than $p < 0.05$, the accepted standard for "statistical significance", which is portrayed in common parlance as a new "fact". These images or metaphors really may change how we treat an individual patient in front of us.

Doctors have, I think, always been empiricists, even the purgers and cuppers, the Brunonians[13] who used heroic doses and the Hahnemannians who used the infinitesimally small ones of the homeopathic religion, and the folk practitioners described by Keith Thomas,[14] Roy Porter[15] or Mark Twain.[16] Science, of course, gained the upper hand historically and scientific rationalism was opposed to religious authority.

## The philosophy of medicine and Polanyi

When I came to the study of the philosophy of medicine, I became concerned at the notion that no knowledge existed outside the ring fence of the physical sciences. Second, I came to believe that a grounding in medical epistemology was important to the study of medical ethics. Insofar as doctors could be described as belonging to any philosophical position, it seemed to be positivism and I wasn't happy with that. There seemed to me to be a need to connect the personal, the experience of people and about people, with the world of our admittedly incomplete trials. And to do so with rigour. It was Michael Polanyi – whose greatest work, *Personal Knowledge*, was published nearly 50 years ago – who seemed to say something relevant, new and important. Polanyi belonged to a group of great scientists that emerged from Hungary in the early 20th century. Originally trained as a doctor, he became a physical chemist, corresponding with Einstein and anticipating discoveries which later gained others the award of a Nobel Prize. Yet he is remembered for his philosophical writings, always grounded in his experience as a practising scientist. In these, he argues that we can reconnect science and the humanities; that personal participation and imagination are *essentially* involved in both science and the humanities and that meanings created in the sciences are no closer to reality than meanings created in the arts, moral judgements or religion. These meanings are of no greater or lesser importance through the presence or absence of personal participation and imagination.

In Polanyi's theory of personal knowledge the processes of knowing (and therefore of science) are rooted throughout, from our selection of a problem to the verification of a discovery, in personal acts of tacit integration, not in explicit operations of logic.

Its method is not detachment but involvement; not scepticism but belief in the coherence and meaning in things.

Margery Grene[17] comments that the selection of a problem takes us back to Plato's *Meno*:

> Why, on what lines will you look, Socrates, for a thing of whose nature you know nothing at all? Pray, what sort of thing, amongst those that you know not, will you treat us to as the object of your search? Or even supposing, at the best, that you hit upon it, how will you know it is the thing you did not know?

## The nature of knowledge

If we are committed to the belief that all cognitive acts are wholly explicit, then we can only know what is capable of being verbalised or is plainly at the centre of our attention. From this perspective, Meno's question is puzzling. Polanyi's view suggests instead that we must admit into the very nature of mind the kind of groping that constitutes the recognition of a problem. If we move from considering knowledge of a problem to knowledge of a skill, an example will make this clear. I may know perfectly well how to play the piano or how to ride a bicycle or how to palpate the spleen but I am unable to articulate the particulars of what I know explicitly. Indeed, if I attempted to concentrate on the particulars of those acts, I would become incapable of accomplishing them at all. The pianist who concentrates on the individual finger movement ceases to play; indeed, few can describe exactly what constitutes "touch". But the particulars are not specifiable. One doesn't learn to play the piano or to ride a bicycle or palpate the spleen by learning a series of particulars. In fact, we can't even say what they are. Ask the average pianist or cyclist or clinician! The principle by which a cyclist keeps his balance is not generally known.[18] This unspecifiable part of knowledge is left unsaid, even in principle.

Plato says that to search for the solution is an absurdity: for either you know what you are looking for, in which case there is no problem, or you don't know what you're looking for, so you can't expect to find anything or recognise it. Knowledge of a problem, like the knowledge of unspecifiables, is a knowing of more than I can tell. To see a problem is to have an intimation of hitherto not comprehended particulars. The theory of tacit knowing establishes a meaningful relationship between two terms: *from* the proximal and subsidiary *to* the distal and focal. Tacit knowing is the understanding of the comprehensive entity which these two terms jointly constitute.

We see the same logical structure in the body–mind relation as in the relation between clues and the image to which the clues point. We observe external objects by being subsidiarily aware of the impact they make on our bodies and of the responses our bodies make to them. All our conscious transactions with the world involve the subsidiary use of our bodies. Active consciousness achieves coherence by integrating clues to the things on which they bear or integrating parts to the wholes they form. One level of awareness is for clues and one for the focally apprehended comprehensive entity to which these elements point. Subsidiary elements lose their functional appearance when we stop looking *from* them and look *at* them, in themselves. We know a comprehensive entity by interiorising its parts or making ourselves dwell in them.

To make this clearer, one example that Polanyi gives is taken from perception. Consider a blind man using a stick. Its impact on his hand is transformed as he learns to use it. It becomes a sentient extension of his own body, as its point touches the objects he is exploring; it has been interiorised. The proximal particulars of impacts on his hand are tacitly known as he concentrates on the distal focus of the objects he explores. He dwells in the stick.

> Our awareness of our body for attending to things outside it suggests a wider generalisation of the feeling we have of our body. Whenever we use certain things for attending *from* them to other things, in the way in which we always use our own body, these things change their appearance. They appear to us now in terms of the entities to which we are attending *from* them, just as we feel our own body in terms of the things outside to which we are attending *from* our body. In this sense we can say that when we make a thing function as the proximal term of tacit knowing, we incorporate it in our body – or extend our body to include it – so that we come to dwell in it.[19]

Indwelling is the proper means of knowing man and the humanities. Aesthetic appreciation, for example, may be represented as the entering into a work of art and thus dwelling in the mind of its creator. Our ways of knowing things in science and of appreciating things in art are essentially similar.

Humanities are not something added on to science, but part of a common culture.

A biologist, a doctor, an art dealer, and a cloth merchant acquire their expert knowledge in part from text books but these texts are no use without the accompanying training of the senses, by which they acquire the right sense or feel for identifying a certain biological specimen, the symptoms of a certain sickness, a genuine master painting or a distinctive quality fabric. An acknowledged expert is believed to *know* whether such things fulfil the standards of good specimens of their own kind. Such knowledge is the fruit of a long reflective experience or acquired by an apprentice to a recognised master. Medicine is full of examples of such knowledge: for example, in the way a clinician will know what is appropriate for a particular patient.[20]

The bearing of medical science, or any other natural science, on the facts of experience is much more specific than that of mathematics, religion or the various humanities. It is justifiable therefore to speak of the verification of science by experience in a sense that would not apply to other articulate systems. The process by which systems other than science (aesthetics, law, religion) are tested and finally accepted may be called, by contrast, a process of validation. To quote Polanyi:[21] our personal participation is, in general, greater in a validation than a verification. The emotional coefficient of assertion is intensified as we pass from the sciences to neighbouring domains of thought. But both verification and validation are everywhere an acknowledgement of a commitment: they claim the presence of something real and external to the speaker. Personal knowledge involves intellectual commitment. As such it is inherently hazardous; that is, our belief in the reality of our insight can be false. Intellectual passions thus have a strong aesthetic aspect.[22] Polanyi defined intellectual passions as:

> a complex system of emotional responses by which scientific value and ingenuity... are appreciated... A scientific theory which calls attention to its own beauty, and partly relies on it for claiming to represent empirical reality, is akin to a work of art... In teaching its own kind of formal excellence science functions like... other constituents of culture.[23]

In purchasing works for the public gallery or making laws or in religious worship we are not engaged in a purely private matter. By contrast, *subjective* experiences can be said only to be authentic and authenticity does not involve a commitment in the sense in which verification and validation do.

Biology is immeasurably rich in things we know and cannot tell. To start with, we know persons. We know them as individuals: persons are fully individual with their own active intelligible coherence, yet also members of the human race. But we cannot devise a definition to specify unambiguously the range over which the human shape may vary. Instead we tacitly integrate subsidiary particulars into a focal whole. We recognise individuals by an empathy or indwelling – by the kind of power used to generate a focal awareness of a comprehensive entity from a subsidiary awareness of its parts. Neurology assumes that the functioning of the nervous system can be reduced to the laws of physics and chemistry and that these determine all the workings that we normally attribute to the mind of an individual. Similarly, psychology reduces its subject matter to establishing explicit relationships between measurable variables. But neither model can account for the unspecifiable propensities of the subject. To know a sane person is to establish a reciprocal relation with him or her. However valuable the sciences of neurology and psychology have been, it is the humanities that remind us that the mechanistic model is not enough. Indeed, even mainstream intellectual disciplines such as neurology have an essential personal component. When we record a patient's reflexes, we are rightly claiming for ourselves powers of personal judgement that are absent in the faculties we are examining in the patient.

## Personal knowledge

Personal knowledge, according to Polanyi, then, has a triadic structure. It requires (1) the act of a person to (2) integrate *from* the subsidiary particulars (3) *to* the focal target – sometimes abbreviated as "from-to" knowing. The process of tacit integration is unspecifiable, the grounds on which knowledge is held to be true are indeterminate, the rules for establishing true and not illusory coherence are unspecifiable and the bearing of empirical knowledge on reality is indeterminate. Personal knowledge means that I must understand the world from my point of view as a person claiming originality and exercising my personal judgement responsibly and with universal intent. The objectivist emphasis on deductive certainties cannot be maintained. In medicine, the soil of our mental development, steeped in the humanities, is the internal and subjective pole of our knowing and validates the facts of our experience. Natural sciences, connoting objectivity, represent the external pole and are mainly responsible for the verification of the facts of experience.

We take our personal participation in the humanities almost for granted: we believe this picture or this piece of music, this poem or (even) this philosophy to be important or beautiful or to hold intimations of an as yet unappreciated reality. Science is not so different even if the personal component is smaller. What Polanyi expounded in detail was perhaps suggested by George Eliot when she wrote:

> [E]ven strictly measuring science could hardly have got on without that forecasting ardour which feels the agitations of discovery beforehand, and has a faith in its preconception that surmounts many failures of experiment. And in relation to human motives and action, passionate belief may have a fuller efficacy. Here enthusiasm may have the validity of proof, and... give the type of what will one day be general... Men may dream in demonstrations, and cut an illusory world in the shape of axioms, definitions and propositions, with a final exclusion of fact signed Q.E.D. No formulas for thinking will save us mortals from mistake in our imperfect apprehension of the matter to be thought about. And since the unemotional intellect may carry us into a mathematical dreamland where nothing is but what is not, perhaps an emotional intellect may have absorbed into its passionate vision of possibilities some truth of what will be – the more comprehensive massive life feeding theory with new material, as the sensibility of the artist seizes combinations which science explains and justifies. At any rate presumptions to the contrary are not to be trusted. We must be patient with the inevitable makeshift of our human thinking, whether in its sum total or in the separate minds that have made the sum. Columbus had some impressions about himself which we call superstitions, and used some arguments which we disapprove; but he had also some true physical conceptions, and he had the passionate patience of genius to make them tell on mankind. The world has made up its mind rather contemptuously about those who were deaf to Columbus.[24]

Drusilla Scott[25] comments that in the play of *Everyman* he had a friend called Five Wits. This name indicated the five senses of Everyman but it might also include all the inarticulate powers inherited from our evolutionary history. It seems agreeable to think of Five Wits as Everyman's dog. In the Everyman play, Five Wits was disparaged as a useless, unreliable creature while knowledge was commended by the priests as Everyman's true friend. And now, Five Wits is disparaged again, for science mistrusts these unregulated powers. If we are to account for creative discovery, we need Five Wits. Without his powers of tacit knowing, no discovery would be possible. The priests also taught that Fellowship was a worthless rascally friend to Everyman. Science ignores him. But truth can only be pursued in a Society of Explorers. Fellowship comes back to go with Everyman on his quest. We must explore meaning together. Man lives in the meanings he is able to discern. Although Bishop Butler's common sense told him that everything is what it is and not another thing, our experiences with illusions breed a common sense that knows that everything is not always what it "is", i.e. what it *seems* to us to be. So we cannot avoid resorting to personal judgement to decide when something is what it is. And, as we have seen, our personal judgement is what *it* is because of the clues we dwell in, including, of course, the general views to which we are committed about the nature of things and the nature of knowledge. As to validity in art, truth in myths, the possibility of theism or the relevance of all this to a free society, I must leave those to the reader's intellectual curiosity and future reading, for which Polanyi's *Meaning* is as good a start as any other.[26]

# References and notes

1   McManus IC. Humanity and the medical humanities. *Lancet* 1995; **346**: 1143–5.
2   Dickens C. *Hard Times*. Bradbury & Evans, 1854.
3   Williams R. *Monmouth Diocesan Newsletter* 1998; **121**:5.
4   Pellegrino ED. Educating the humanist physician. An ancient ideal reconsidered. *JAMA* 1974; **227**: 1288–94.
5   Clouser KD. Humanities and the medical school: a sketched rationale and description. *Br J Med Educ* 1971; **5**: 226–31.
6   Steiner G. *In Bluebeard's Castle: some notes towards the re-definition of culture.* London: Faber and Faber, 1971.
7   Snow CP. *The Two Cultures and the Scientific Revolution*. The Rede Lecture. Cambridge: Cambridge University Press, 1959.
8   Glymour C, Stalker D. Engineers, cranks, physicians, magicians. *N Engl J Med* 1983; **308**: 960–4.
9   Hampton JR. The end of medical history? *J Roy Coll Physicians London* 1998; **32**: 366–75.
10  Naylor CD. Grey zones of clinical practice: some limits to evidence based

medicine. *Lancet* 1995; **345**: 840–2.

11  Charlton BG. Book review of evidence-based medicine. *J Eval Clin Pract* 1997; **3**: 169–72.

12  McGouran R. What price prevention? *Hospital Doctor* 1997: April 3: 12.

13  Guthrie D. *A History of Medicine.* London: T. Nelson and Sons, 1945.

14  Thomas K. *Religion and the Decline of Magic.* London: Weidenfeld and Nicolson,1971.

15  Porter R. *The Greatest Benefit to Mankind.* London: HarperCollins, 1997.

16  Whorton JC. Traditions of folk medicine in America. *JAMA* 1987; **257**:1632–5.

17  Grene M. *The Knower and the Known.* Berkeley: University of California Press, 1974.

18  Polanyi M. *Personal Knowledge.* London: Routledge and Kegan Paul, 1958: 49 *et seq.*

19  Polanyi M. *The Tacit Dimension.* London: Routledge and Kegan Paul, 1967: 21 *et seq.* See also Polanyi M. Tacit knowing: its bearing on some problems of philosophy. In: Grene M (ed.). *Knowing and Being.* London: Routledge and Kegan Paul, 1969.

20  Epstein RM. Mindful practice. *JAMA* 1999; **282**: 833–9.

21  Polanyi[18], 202.

22  Jha SR. The tacit-explicit connection: Polanyian integrative philosophy and a neo-Polanyian medical epistemology. *Theoretical Med Bioethics* 1998; **19**: 547–68.

23  Polanyi[18], 133.

24  Eliot G. *Daniel Deronda.* London: Blackwood, 1876.

25  Scott D. *Michael Polanyi.* London: SPCK, 1996.

26  Polanyi M, Prosch H. *Meaning.* Chicago: University of Chicago Press, 1975.

# 15

# The humanities' role in improving health and clinical care

Richard Edwards

At a time when objective evidence-based healthcare is the priority, it can be argued that specific consideration needs to be given to the subjective, human aspects of care. The recreational and therapeutic potential of participation in the humanities, as represented by art therapy, music therapy, dance therapy, and therapeutic creative writing,[1,2] has been described elsewhere.

However, three other aspects of the important relationship between medicine and the humanities can be considered. They have practical implications for the future practice of medicine and delivery of healthcare.

## The humanities as a resource: the expression of human experiences and emotions

They present a wealth of recorded human experiences and emotions in a wide range of life situations. Some of these are imagined whilst others take life experiences and are descriptively fashioned by creative talent and skill. These descriptions allow professionals to recognise, and acknowledge emotions both in the patient and their family as well as in themselves. Such emotions are increasingly recognised as important determinants of health and of a successful response to treatment.

## The humanities as a means of helping communication

Sharing the meanings of words, images, concepts, and emotions is an essential component of successful communication between care givers and the cared-for patients and their families. Those meanings derive from actual or imaginary shared experiences and emotions; their expression may help explain how an individual copes with the uncertainty of illness and its outcomes.

## The humanities as an attitudinal resource in healthcare professional education

Adding the "medical humanities" as yet another speciality, discipline or subject into already overcrowded curricula is impractical and unlikely to be successful. It is far better to employ published narratives or artistic representations of ill health as qualitative input alongside actual patients' narrative,[3] to widen perspective and facilitate a more sympathetic understanding of the "human condition". Such understanding could lead to improved communication between healthcare professionals and with patients and their families and ameliorate arrogant, ignorant or insensitive attitudes. The personal insight the student gains can also be a valuable resource to help young people cope with the stresses of their academic and professional lives.

# Is anything needed beyond evidence-based healthcare?

Why should a physician be concerned about possible relationships between medicine and the humanities? Porter[4] suggests that 20th century medicine was a victim of its own success and that the expectations created in the patients and public are, like all consumer demand, destined to be unsatisfied. Illich[5] has eloquently argued the harms of the "medicalisation" of current social problems. However, the current view is that modern medicine makes a large contribution to health, while the social environment is a second, separate determinant of health and well-being in society.[6]

Today's high spending on healthcare has not resulted in people feeling better about themselves or society. This may reflect a search for something beyond science, into the spiritual and existential domain. It may also represent a cynicism about current evaluated medicine, which has lost some of the magic and mystery of ancient remedies. The use of unproven "alternative" therapies has burgeoned and the media appear to fuel the trend of confusion between facts and fiction in health issues.

Reductionist science is immensely successful in analysing disease in ever greater mechanistic detail. Thus, it is easy for the patient's "dis-ease" to receive less attention than his or her "disease", though such "dis-ease" (or other manifestation of psychosomatic medicine) may underlie increasing dependence on healthcare services.[7] Reductionist science can provide facts to inform decision making but these facts must be understood and felt to be relevant to the individual, if they are to understand and use information in decision making.

It is patently obvious that it is impossible (and is likely to remain impossible) to have "gold standard" scientific evidence from equally rigorous research studies directly relevant to each and every patient in each and every possible situation. The movement of evidence-based healthcare has been urgently needed, but it will be found wanting because it is difficult to match the results from studies of large populations to the situation of an individual. Even in ideal circumstances, when appropriate evidence is available to both healthcare professional and patient and both understand and accept the evidence, it remains imperative to address and respond sympathetically to the emotional consequences of the diagnosis or treatment.

An assertion of this chapter is that study of the humanities in their various forms may provide valuable opportunities to bridge the "organism – mechanisms" divide. This becomes particularly important if due respect is to be given to self and self-determination, as they seem to have increasing importance for health.[8] Moreover, the sharing of mutually agreed expectations from healthcare services may help to restore some trust in the relationship of healthcare professionals with patients and the public (Fig. 15.1).

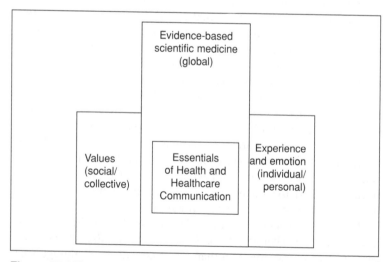

**Figure 15.1** The (objective) nature of scientific evidence is reinterpreted through the values of society and the individual's previous experiences, to influence their personal handling of disease and its treatment.

# The humanities as a resource: the expression of human experiences and emotions

The psychologist Carl Jung described shared "archetypes" or ideas, based on generic societal experience, which influence human beliefs and behaviours.[9] What then are the humanities (or in this context the medical humanities)? What is health? How can it be improved? What constitutes a shared understanding of health issues? For the purposes of this chapter the humanities are considered (if not specifically defined) as the promotion and study of the visual, literary, and performance arts, but influences of design and historical writings should not be excluded from a broader definition. In Wales the humanities are celebrated at the National Eisteddfod, where prominence is given to newly created prose, art, vocal and instrumental music, dance, and poetry. The humanities can be considered in the wider context of the influence of science, architecture, and politics on the social fabric and topography of the country, so that the definition of the humanities must extend well beyond the boundaries of what is taught at universities.

---

## Humanities: communicating health ideas, images and emotions

- Literature – fiction and poetry are qualitative records of perceptions of health, disease, and death, sharing the emotional interpretations across the generations.
- History – formal analyses of sociohistorical context of medical and healthcare developments.
- Music – may be an expression of emotion, appreciation/enjoyment/or as part of music therapy; cognitive neuropsychology.
- Dance – can reflect mood and is appreciated, enjoyed or used in dance therapy to ensure exercise and co-ordination and re-education in rehabilitation.
- Philosophy/theology/religion – search for meaning, purpose, and "soul-fulfilment" beyond healthcare.

---

I have no formal or professional affiliations with the humanities, but know the lifelong restorative benefits of their intellectual and spiritual resources. This analysis represents a well-meaning (though "amateur" in the true sense of the word) attempt to integrate the "truths of science" with the insights and environmental influences of the humanities: the aim is to improve both the quality of healthcare delivery and the fundamental health of the population.

The first proposition is that an exploration of the emotional content of key events and life experiences must be communicated to those involved in trying to promote health or manage disease in an individual patient. The personal meaning of the "experiences" of a person, whether real or acquired through reading, film or television, can inform the clinical relationship and thus make decision making more appropriate to an individual's circumstance.

# The humanities as a means of helping communication: sharing individual feelings and experience

NHS Wales, in its 1998 White Paper *Putting Patients First*,[10] commits all parts of the NHS in Wales to contribute to achieving the seven core values in the effective and efficient delivery of healthcare (see box). These corporate "societal" values are clearly essential for successful healthcare delivery. However, the humanity of the care itself depends on the extent to which carer and cared-for can empathise, i.e. share experiences and/or feelings about the significance of the illness. Disease-specific voluntary support groups have usually come together because they share mutual feelings of fear and hope, have common experiences of symptoms and treatments and are motivated to help others avoid some of the anxieties they have experienced.

---

### Values and emotional states important in communicating health issues

| *Societal – core values* | *Individual – experience/ feelings/states* |
|---|---|
| Fairness | Fear/anxiety |
| Effectiveness | Sadness/depression |
| Efficiency | Endurance/courage/resilience |
| Responsiveness | Expectation/reassurance/hope |
| Integration | Acceptability/equanimity |
| Accountability | Self-confidence/respect |
| Flexibility | Healing/cure |

---

There appear to be two "currencies" already in existence in healthcare. One determines society's acceptance of its obligations to care. The other currency determines the successful communication between professionals and patients. The humanities may provide quasi-historical or academic insights into these influences. Their great strength is that they provide ways in which people can communicate.[11,12] Patients thereby have a "language" with which they can share feelings and handle uncertainty. Fiction may be effective as it explores the possible consequences of differing courses of action. The explanation of personal feelings through fictional stories allows the patient to rehearse possible consequences. The importance of the medical humanities is not antagonistic to the current drive towards evidence-based healthcare delivery; it is an essential component within an integrated healthcare service, which deserves to be researched appropriately.

It is important to avoid the cynical misinterpretation that all organisational interventions in healthcare have their origin in the need to save money. What price a smile, a kind word of sympathy, reassurance or explanation? Corporate values are reflected in the way staff behave. They cannot be imposed or purchased *per se*, yet human warmth profoundly alters the patient's experience. Establishing a valid "language" for communication of issues of emotion and experience is important. These expressions of warmth and human values in traditional care-giving cannot become systematised, professionalised and audited without risking all the unwanted consequences foreseen by Illich.[5] It is therefore necessary to have an environment which is rich in different forms of communication and expression of feelings, such as music, art, sculpture, and literature, which can remind or paint an imaginary picture of better times. Heart-warming memories can restore hope to those who may feel they are becoming worthless through age or infirmity. Such "remembered wellness" has been described by Benson[13] and may also be the way the olfactory memories and "relaxation" are induced by aromatherapy, just as music can powerfully recreate an atmosphere. There is a real difference between communicating by sharing memories of enjoyed literature, touch, smell or music and the situation when the same complementary therapies are presented as "proven facts" and expected to correct a wide range of disorders of visceral function underlying ill health. When both patient and professional know the nature of an evoked memory, the conversation is a vehicle for communicating deeper feelings; when the evoked sensation is perceived as part of a "curative" process the expectations are unreal and based on falsehood.

This argument does not undermine or question unthinkingly the validity of complementary (alternative) therapies, but it seeks to distinguish between whether or not the therapy is effective. This is a matter for formal randomised controlled trials, as in the case of evidence of successful treatment of asthma,[14] and studies of how the complementary therapy achieves its effects. Evidence-based healthcare is rationally founded on reproducible, fully accountable evidence. This is not the case for the complementary (alternative) therapies, which are founded on complex belief systems and explanatory "stories". Yet evidence-based healthcare needs to recognise the popularity of the alternative therapies[15] as patients and public seek more than existing scientifically based healthcare has to offer. It is possible that several things are being sought, amongst them:

- buying time and "hands on" contact
- stories that can be believed to help give meaning to symptom concerns and treatments offered
- stories that can be believed to provide hope of cure, when the honest imparting of information by conventional healthcare professionals has heralded mortality
- control over when the "therapy" is used.

Clearly, evidence-based healthcare needs to take notice of this and to seek to provide better, more understandable "stories" based on scientific evidence,[16,17] to provide time for these to be discussed and to co-ordinate care among all members of the multiprofessional team.[18]

Throughout the ages the *gwerin* (ordinary working people) of Wales have faced many and varied adversities. They have often transcended them through a passionate commitment to poetry, literature, and music, shared socially within a stable framework of church and chapel life and local and regional *eisteddfodau*. These local cultural festivals across Wales for children and adults ultimately feed talent into the National Eisteddfod. It was through success in the Eisteddfod that quarry workers, coal miners, and tradesmen gained fame (and their work preserved in history) far beyond their material wealth or formal education. Poverty was no bar and the benefits of having such a purpose in life were, and still are, obvious. Today, the health consequences of inequality, unemployment, and "early retirement" have revealed that a sense of purpose or meaning in life is relevant to society's concept of health and the likely demands on healthcare services.

It has been said that a poor man is not someone without money but one without a dream. Another way of saying this is that in contemporary society each and every one of us needs to echo the expressions of the two Martin Luthers: "Here stand I..." (Martin Luther 1483–1546) and "I have a dream..." (Martin Luther King 1929-1968).

## Stories from the humanities

The Bible is the most easily accessible and ancient library which can be read as literature. As such, it is an example of how literature can create images and communicate emotions to help in overcoming life challenges[19] and disease suffered, perhaps in a way which is more meaningful to the sufferer and family than a purely factual clinical diagnosis, prognosis, and treatment plan.

The philosopher Ludwig Wittgenstein (1889–1951) believed that the limits of thought are determined by the limits of expression of those thoughts, i.e. words and language.[20]

Words are also important for communication of meaning and mental images of illness, disease processes, health, and hope. The Bible itself relates descriptions of many key life experiences and emotions, equally relevant today as in the time they were written. A simple "telephone directory" exercise to trace words in the Bible is of little value, unless the contexts of those words are also considered. The box illustrates that health and emotional issues are as important today as two millennia ago, and also that many references are to words that convey reassurance and hope.

It cannot escape comment that the current decline of religious beliefs and practices may be of relevance to health. Formerly, chapels and churches provided some of the support and reassurance sought today from healthcare services. The search for equanimity continues as in past ages. Izaak Walton (1593–1683) in his celebrated book *The Compleat Angler* encouraged his reader to be grateful for health and to value it next to a "good conscience". It is significant that he considered health to be secondary to "good conscience" as a blessing. It was, and probably still is, a blessing beyond that which money can buy. Good health underlies the primacy of peace of mind, which constitutes a mental attitude to health and disease; this may be what Walton terms a "good conscience".

# Health-related references from Holy Scripture

*Life state*
| | |
|---|---|
| birth/born | 135 |
| child/youth | 187 |
| old/age | 329 |
| die/death/dead | 781 |

*Experience/emotion*
| | |
|---|---|
| grief/grieve/mourn | 74 |
| suffering/pain/anguish | 45 |
| sorrow/sad/despair/guilt | 107 |
| fear/afraid | 514 |
| disease/affliction(afflict★) | 162 |

*Individual identity*
| | |
|---|---|
| soul | 328 |
| self/person | 62 |

*Healthcare/remedies*
| | |
|---|---|
| comfort | 59 |
| cure/heal/forgive(forgiv★) | 114 |
| health | 17 |
| medicine | 2 |
| physician | 6 |
| midwife | 3 |

*Reassurance/healing*
| | |
|---|---|
| hope | 109 |
| save (excluding usage meaning "except") | 1288 |
| salvation | 140 |
| spirit | 361 |

There is only one reference to "doctor" and that is to Gameliel the teacher of Paul, who is noted as a Doctor of Law. There is no mention of depression or melancholy. Healing may perhaps be seen in these ancient writings as a quest for equanimity as in "heal my soul" (*Psalm* 41:4), "time to heal" (*Ecclesiastes* 3.3) and "heal the broken hearted" (*Luke* 4:18). There is a metaphorical description of the stages of life from childhood to old age presented in *Ecclesiastes* 12: 1–8. In the Apocrypha there is advice to "Honour a Physician" (*Ecclesiasticus* 38).

# The humanities as possible components of professional, medical and healthcare education

Moran Campbell argued that more important than the "stories" of basic science in medical education is the incorporation of the scientific method in order to develop what the philosopher Karl Popper referred to as the "searchlight" rather than the "bucket" function of the mind.[21] The stimulation of a questioning approach is seen in problem-based learning, where the humanities can be an important resource. This searchlight on the humanity content of professional care practices can promote reflective practice and learning. Albert Einstein asserted that the imagination is more important than knowledge; the ability to think and question creatively can inform the research questions which explore the complexities of the human condition in health and disease.

The public hears stories about health scares in profusion. Medicine and other healthcare professions are no longer seen as vocations similar to a priesthood. The information revolution has challenged the previous sacred image of professionals. Yet this is not a recent phenomenon: Bernard Shaw in his play *The Doctor's Dilemma*[22] elucidated the tension between health policies and therapeutic practices. Another play by Shaw called *The Apple Cart*,[23] the novel *The Citadel* by AJ Cronin[24] and Henrik Ibsen's play *An Enemy of the People*[25] similarly provide images and rhetoric with which to reflect on the direction, quality and mode of delivery of healthcare today.

Literary images of lasting importance can convey the poignancy of the human condition and are used in the modern integrated medical curriculum described earlier in this volume (Chapter 9). For example, in Oscar Wilde's *The Picture of Dorian Gray* is the statement that the "tragedy of old age is not that one is old, but one is young".[26] This eloquent statement could provide a thought-provoking examination essay question to be discussed in relation to care of the elderly, perhaps coupled with interpretation of the richly metaphorical descriptions of the ages of man as presented two centuries BC in *Ecclesiastes* (12:1–8). Similarly, the experience of terminal illness and approaching death might be compared to the account given in *The Death of Ivan Illyich* by Tolstoy a century ago.[27] Hysterical conversion disorders, hypochondriasis and Munchausen's syndrome could be contrasted with the problems of imagined ill health described by Molière in the 18th century in *The Imaginary Invalid*,[28] or in Frances Hodgson Burnett's children's story *The Secret Garden*,[29] in which a child invalid is restored to health by a change in illness belief and involvement in tending a secret garden. The poetry of Dylan Thomas, "And death shall have no dominion" and "Do not go gentle into that good night," evokes powerful images and emotions which may be used to inspire interest in the social or psychological aspects of care. These books are easily available but time to read is at a premium. When choosing what to read, the words of Mark Twain should not be forgotten: "The man who does not read good books has no advantage over the man who can't read them".

The obvious benefits of purpose in life are nowhere more evident than in the fascinating account of *The Surgeon of Crowthorne*,[30] a mentally disturbed man who contributed to the mammoth task of compiling the *Oxford English Dictionary* a hundred years ago. The author raises the important question of whether today's drug therapy would have prevented this dedicated commitment to reading, writing and collating information for the dictionary. Many contemporary accounts of great composers and authors speculate about relationships between psychology, psychopathology and artistic creativity[31] and this debate is likely to continue. It would be a doubtful achievement of modern society if, through the well-meaning treatment of all "medicalised" distressing, painful, non-conformist mental states or personal characteristics, future peaks and troughs of artistic or scientific creative talent were smoothed to mediocre conformity.

## The humanities: their purpose and meaning as important to health

A Native American chief wrote: "There is a longing in the heart of my people to reach out and grasp that which is needed for our survival. There is a longing among the young of my nation to secure for themselves and their people the skills that will provide them with a sense of worth and purpose".[32] This may be echoed by many peoples of the world today.

The humanities are important records of communal experience in dealing with life's challenges and are a resource to develop coping strategies and enrich life. Whether related directly or indirectly to healthcare, appreciation of the humanities is a potentially valuable source of purpose and fulfilment in life for individuals and communities. As such, the humanities are becoming increasingly relevant to a society in which the pursuit of health and consumer expectations make great demands on healthcare services, despite "biomedicine" (as Kleinman[33] defines current western medicine) playing an ever more prominent role in healthcare expenditure.

The current aim for sustainable health is integral to the context of sustainable community development in Wales. There are important precedents, such as the Llangollen International Musical Eisteddfod in the small Welsh town of my childhood, the peripatetic National Eisteddfod of Wales and the legendary successes of book selling at Hay-on-Wye,[34] which led to the internationally known Hay Literary Festival. While none has any declared direct health connections, they are implicitly powerful in fostering cultural activities, thereby directing attention away from symptoms of ill health (i.e. what my wife Eleri, a physiotherapist, calls the "distraction principle") towards fulfilment of individual aspiration and achievement in ways which improve self-confidence. This is not far removed from the importance of valuing "self" and "self-determination" as contributors to health. Wales, like other small nations, must not fall into the trap of believing solely in an economic salvation for its social and personal ills. The cultural inspiration and social energy of the humanities is most definitely an asset, which may have a valuable influence on the future success of Wales!

The 20th century has seen the phenomenal power of science for good and for harm. Science is now an inevitable component of our history and thus our humanity. It would be as sad an oversight if humanity were to be excluded from our science as if science were to be excluded from our consideration of the social context of the humanities.

These personal reflections have been in the spirit of the recommendations of the General Medical Council,[35] for reform of medical education. They resonate with one of the aims of *Medical Humanities*,[36] a new journal published by the British Medical Journal Publishing Group.

The humanities can redress the balance, create better visions of health and social contentment and resist the manipulation of healthcare for political gain. The qualitative aspects of science and medicine can only be explored through the language and images provided by the humanities, making investment in qualitative research methodology an essential prerequisite to developing a healthier society, whose prosperity can be maintained.

# References and notes

1   Greenhalgh T. Writing as therapy: effects on immune mediated illness need substantiation in independent studies. *BMJ* 1999; **319**: 270–1.
2   Bolton G. *The Therapeutic Potential of Creative Writing*. London: Jessica Kingsley, 1999.
3   Greenhalgh T, Hurwitz B. Why study narrative? *BMJ* 1999; **318**: 48–50.
4   Porter R. *The Greatest Benefit to Mankind: a medical history of humanity from antiquity to the present*. London: HarperCollins, 1997: 710–18.
5   Illich I. *Limits to medicine. Medical Nemesis: the expropriation of health*. Harmondsworth: Penguin Books, 1976.
7   Shorter E. *From Paralysis to Fatigue: a history of psychosomatic illness in the modern era*. New York: Freedom Press, 1992.
8   Corin E. The social and cultural matrix of health and disease. In: Evans RG, Barer ML, Marmor TR (eds). *Why Are Some People Healthy and Others Not?* New York: Aldine De Gruyter, 1994: 93–129.
9   Jacobi J. *The Psychology of CG Jung*, 7th edn. London: Routledge and Kegan Paul, 1968.
10  NHS Wales. *Putting Patients First*. Cardiff: Welsh Office, 1998.
11  Asher R. The medical education of the patient and the public. In: Avery Jones F (ed.). *Talking Sense*. London: Churchill Livingstone, 1986: 102–10.
12  Fletcher C, Peeling P. *Talking and Listening to Patients: a modern approach*. London: Nuffield Provincial Hospitals Trust, 1988.
13  Benson H. *Timeless Healing: the power and biology of belief*. London: Simon and Schuster, 1996.
14  Reilly DT, Taylor MA, McSharry C, Aitchinson T. Is homeopathy a placebo response? A controlled trial of homeopathic immunotherapy (HIT) in atopic asthma. *Complement Therap Med* 1993; **1**: 24–5.
15  Eisenberg DM, Davis RB, Ettner SL *et al.* Trends in alternative medicine use in the United States, 1990–1997: results of a follow-up national survey. *JAMA* 1998; **280**: 1569–75.
16  Foundation for Integrated Medicine. *Integrated Healthcare: a way forward for the next five years?* London: Prince of Wales Initiative on Integrated Medicine, 1997.
17  Jonas WB. Alternative medicine – learning from the past, examining the present, advancing the future. *JAMA* 1998; **280**: 1616–18.
18  Edwards RHT. Time for sharing responsibility. *J Roy Coll Physicians London* 1999; **33**: 145–7.
19  World Library. *The Bible: a multimedia experience*. Irvine, California: Softkey, 1995.
20  Honderich T. *The Oxford Companion to Philosophy*. Oxford: Oxford University Press, 1995: 912–16.
21  Campbell EJM. Basic science, science and medical education. *Lancet* 1976; **i**: 134–6.

22  Shaw GB. *The Doctor's Dilemma: a tragedy*. Harmondsworth: Penguin, 1946.

23  Shaw GB. *The Apple Cart*. Harmondsworth: Penguin, 1956.

24  Cronin AJ. *The Citadel*. London: Gollancz, 1937.

25  Ibsen H. *An Enemy of the People*. London: Eyre Methuen, 1980.

26  Wilde O. *The Picture of Dorian Gray*. London: Minster Classics, 1968: 337.

27  Tolstoy L. *The Death of Ivan Illyich and Other Stories* (trans. R Edmonds). Harmondsworth: Penguin, 1960.

28  Molière JBP. *The Imaginary Invalid* (trans. J Wood). Harmondsworth: Penguin, 1959.

29  Burnett FH. *The Secret Garden*. Harmondsworth: Penguin, 1973.

30  Winchester S. *The Surgeon of Crowthorne*. London: Penguin, 1998.

31  Vernon PE (ed.). *Creativity*. Harmondsworth: Penguin, 1970.

32  George D, Hirnshall H. *My Heart Soars*. Saanichton BC: Hancock House, 1974.

33  Kleinman A. *Writing at the Margin: discourse between anthropology and medicine*. Berkeley: University of California Press, 1995.

34  Booth R, Stuart L. *My Kingdom of Books* Talybont Ceredigion: Y Lolfa, 1999.

35  General Medical Council. *Tomorrow's Doctors: Recommendations on Undergraduate Medical Education*. London: General Medical Council, 1993.

36  Evans M, Greaves D. Exploring the medical humanities: A new journal will explore a new conception of medicine. *BMJ* 1999; 319:1216.

# 16

# Philosophy and the medical humanities

Martyn Evans

## What philosophy is – or might be

Oscar Wilde said of philosophers, no doubt unkindly, that theirs is the "art of bearing up under other people's troubles". I take this to mean that philosophers have supposedly no troubles of their own or at least, not nearly enough troubles to satisfy that particular critic. Whether or not philosophers should feel sensitive to this charge, we might sometimes seem to invite it. The American philosopher Stephen Toulmin – whom I will otherwise applaud, below, in a different context – famously declared that the modern surge of interest in medical ethics would be the saving of moral philosophy.[1] His confident prediction precipitated the swingeing response that medicine was evidently confronted, within its own very house, by "squatting philosophers, looking for work".[2]

The suggestion – and I admit it makes me nervous – seems to be that, lacking authentic problems of our own, philosophers have adopted the perfectly genuine problems of other disciplines or practices such as medicine, staying in business effectively by trading under assumed names or with rebranded goods. I think the charge could be resisted in two ways: first, by pointing to decently authentic philosophical problems and second, by demonstrating the irreducibly philosophical dimensions of practical and theoretical problems in other disciplines, practices or professions, such as medicine.

On the first point, generally speaking, isolated or abstract questions about what constitutes a human *person*, the nature of human experience, the relation between reason and perception, the nature of the ethical life and so on are indeed typically left to philosophers to contemplate; philosophers happily oblige. The second point is, however, more interesting and considerably more far reaching. For such abstract questions have a habit of spilling over into the practical world. It is striking how often this happens in the world of clinical medicine and we might usefully list quite a number of examples, as follows.

When doctors acknowledge a patient's freedom to make "bad" choices seemingly against his or her clinical interests, they acknowledge the trumping of science by ethics and they confront the uneasy blend of the biological and the biographical in the human person. When society sanctions the removal of vital transplant organs from donors with still-beating hearts, it takes up a position on the essentially philosophical question of choosing which point in the processes of human dying will be deemed to count as death. Under mental health law someone can lose his liberty and even be medically treated for his mental condition against his will, if he falls short of a prescribed threshold of rationality to the extent that he is a danger to himself or to others. The law presumes that we understand what rationality is and that we can measure it. The UK "official position" on the moral status of the early human embryo presumes that our ignorance, as to whether a given conceptus will result in none, one or more identifiable human individuals, is a sufficient basis for regarding such an embryo as expendable in the interests of research.

The rationing of socially funded healthcare resources presumes a certain conception of justice, based on maximising the public good at the expense of individual interests. Current efforts at health promotion emphasise an individual's responsibility for health, yet this person lives amidst social and environmental influences beyond their control. Those who seek genetic explanations for undesirable tendencies such as aggressive behaviour are, to say the least, in danger of presuming that human moral choices are shaped by physical mechanisms, leaving free will as little more than a cosy fiction. The pharmacological approach to psychiatry paints an explicitly physicalist picture of the relation between mind and body. And so on.

In short, "other people's troubles" in these contexts are, whether they like it or not, troubles under which philosophers also bear up and have borne up; moreover to the extent that medicine *contemplates* and takes up theoretical positions on questions like these, medicine becomes to that extent philosophical. The list we've just considered shows how rich medicine's philosophical dimensions are.

So doctors and philosophers alike are, I think, justifiably

interested in many of the *ideas* central to both clinical and theoretical medicine. These ideas right now include the widespread suggestion[3, 4] that an understanding of the arts and humanities disciplines offers something important to medical education, practice and research. This suggestion has to an extent emerged in response to some of the "troubles" besetting modern medicine in its science-based but cash-limited form, in particular the charge that scientific medicine is remote, detached, impersonal or – worse – in danger of somehow missing the point with regard to the reasons why patients seek help from doctors.[5] Significantly, the following extract is part of what was a new entry for the fourth edition (1995) of *The Oxford Handbook of Clinical Specialties*.

> When we read alone and for pleasure, our defences are down – and we hide nothing from the great characters of fiction. In our consulting rooms, and on the ward, we so often do our best to hide everything, beneath the white coat, or the avuncular bedside manner. So often, a professional detachment is all that is left after all those years inured to the foibles, fallacies and frictions of our patients' tragic lives. It is at the point where art and medicine collide, that doctors can re-attach themselves to the human race and re-feel those emotions which motivate or terrify our patients. ... *[E]very* contact with patients has an ethical and artistic dimension, as well as a technical one.[6]

This passage confronts, rather strikingly, the question of what medicine is *for*: it highlights the importance of distinguishing and emphasising medicine's nature and goals and of embodying these in the clinical work of the practitioner. Distinguishing the nature and goals of any practice is a philosophical task. By this I do not mean that it is to be left to professional philosophers to attempt it. Rather I mean that anyone trying to elucidate this distinction is engaged in an inescapably philosophical enquiry whether they wish it or not and philosophers (professional and otherwise) have a legitimate interest in that enquiry and, perhaps, a contribution to make.

What might this contribution involve? A difficulty here is that philosophers themselves disagree even over what philosophy actually is, to the extent that Derrida is alleged to be at odds with more traditional philosophers over whether philosophy is possible at all as a discipline distinct from, for instance, literary criticism.[7] But there may be wisdom in more than one view. For instance, David Raphael advertises part of philosophy's dowry as being "the critical examination of assumptions and arguments",[8] which seems self-evidently worthwhile as a procedure for avoiding error, false reasoning or the building of a view upon untenable foundations. Any discipline might adopt this aspect of philosophy for its own more reflective or theoretical aspects; most disciplines do.

Analysis is an essentially *instrumental* form of philosophy. In its most creative aspect it is the exploration of how ideas can work, can collide, what it makes sense to say or to ask, what can constitute an answer to a question. For instance, we may focus on the difference between a question of fact (how many butterflies are there in the room?) and a question of meaning (what should count as a butterfly when we're totalling them up?). Such distinctions are familiar in science and medicine of course. Counting the incidence of a particular medical phenomenon – say, heart attacks – requires the specification of the parameters for "heart attack": these include the criteria which must be fulfilled clinically, pathologically or aetiologically, the allowable variations from the mean in terms of normal (age-related) cardiac function, our confident specification of the observer's competence, the limits of time and place within which observations are to count towards our intended total, and so on. But counting heart attacks also requires that we be in a context in which "heart attack" has *meaning*, which is to say a context in which the idea of a certain distinguishable complex of physical symptoms is recognised as a discrete problem for cardiology. Greaves has shown just how recently that context has emerged in historical terms and just how dependent it remains upon the interplay of scientific and frankly social and cultural factors.[9]

Beyond this instrumental sense lies another and it is more ambitious. Phillips has wryly suggested that we can also think of philosophy in terms of taking seriously the kinds of questions that (at any rate for grown-ups) tend to arise only towards the end of a committed Friday evening at a public house – the "meaning of life" type of question. Philosophers, says Phillips, continue to ponder such questions the following morning, even when sober. (In this, philosophers are enjoined to share the child's sense of wonder at the world's enigmatic and unreasonable nature, according to the advice Sophie receives from her mysterious mentor Albert Knox in Gaarder's best-selling *Sophie's World*.[10]) And indeed, in this more ambitious style, philosophy really does concern the larger and deeper questions about how we are to think about ourselves or about the world around us and our relation to it.

Such questions are officially divided into the categories of *metaphysical* and *epistemological* enquiry with, for good measure, the further and more reassuringly titled category of value enquiry. Between them these categories of questions offer a comprehensive squaring-up of the intellect to the general form of the universe of our human experience. They ask, respectively, what constitutes the world in the most basic sense; how we have knowledge of the world and of ourselves and each other; and how we identify and understand the distinction of some things as being intrinsically desirable or worthwhile. In short, what there *is*, how it's *known*, and why it might be *good*.

Such questions have a grip upon us in the context of trying to understand ourselves; they involve an enquiry into the world that forms part of our enquiry into ourselves. And in this I believe that philosophy and medicine share a common purpose. For medicine is the modern, scientific form of the pursuit of understanding our bodily selves and philosophy is, among other things, the continuing form of the pursuit of understanding our rational and experiential selves. Let me say at once that I do not mean to suggest that our bodily selves are ultimately separable from our rational and experiential selves. Indeed, the suspicion that scientific medicine tends to treat the body as if it were so separable is at the root, I'm sure, of much contemporary criticism of medicine. I mean only that we can distinguish different aspects to our nature as *embodied selves*. It is exceedingly difficult to put this point briefly without seeming obscure. The best I can do here is to say that medicine concerns itself primarily with that embodiment and philosophy primarily with the nature that is thus embodied. How it is that rational beings and bodily creatures are combined in the human constitutes a deep question for both medicine and philosophy. This question is partly medical and partly philosophical, to which any truly rich answer must combine both medical and philosophical insight.

But these are deep waters, deeper than it is possible to venture here. Even without this larger ambition, I hope to have said enough to show that philosophical concerns rise irresistibly in clinical medical practice and to indicate the kinds of thinking that philosophy might bring to bear upon those concerns. To illuminate this more clearly, we can consider the best-recognised connection between medical and philosophical questions, namely the emergence of "medical ethics" as a distinguishable enquiry that properly belongs both clinically at the bedside and reflectively in the study.

# Philosophy and medical ethics

Today a typical reaction to the suggestion that ethics in medicine is a matter of philosophical interest might be to think of something concrete and vivid like the dispute over who is the "real" mother of a child born as a result of a surrogacy arrangement. But ethics has a long history in both medicine and philosophy, and the earliest convergence of medicine and philosophy in ethical matters can be seen in a much more general, diffuse form: such as in Aristotle's suggestion that excellence in human practices such as medicine in itself aligns with *moral* excellence or virtue.[11]

Perhaps we might nowadays be more inclined to distinguish between technical or functional excellence and moral virtue; indeed, the example of functional excellence of highly specialised weaponry seems to demand that we do. But this shows only that ways of thinking about ethics can change. Certainly medicine and philosophy have shared an interest in ethics for more than two millennia.

In reasoning about ethical matters, philosophers have distinguished three forms of interest in the subject. We can distinguish "descriptive ethics", in which one simply notes who says what should or should not be done (as a newspaper report might, for instance), from "normative ethics" in which one goes further and adds one's own opinion (such as a newspaper editorial might). Both of these can be distinguished from a third form of interest, namely "meta-ethics", in which one ponders more abstract questions about the nature of moral judgement itself, perhaps asking exactly what is the force of the word "should" in such a context. A "heavyweight" newspaper might supply even this third kind of concern, in the more reflective of its guest articles.

This threefold distinction is useful in surveying explicitly *medical* ethics as well; indeed it would be surprising if it were not useful, since surely medical ethics is properly thought of as ordinary moral life carried on in a particular context (rather than as some strange and separate species of morality). So a question in "descriptive medical ethics" might be: "What in fact does the BMA say about surrogacy arrangements?", to which the answer can perhaps be found by looking up the appropriate BMA publication. The corresponding question in "normative medical ethics" could be: "What *should* the BMA say about surrogacy arrangements?", a question presumably answered in terms of our own moral opinion on the subject. While "medical meta-ethics" might involve our asking: "What is the source of moral conviction concerning the private arrangements of private citizens?" or, "Why should a doctor's individual choices be constrained by abstract principles attaching to his or her professional or social role?" (Or even "Is an appeal to principles rather than to virtues the best way of analysing moral problems in medical practice?")

Distinguishing among these three kinds of interest in medical ethics questions invites us to consider which ones are the proper concern of philosophers. One view, indeed, actually claims that none of them is. There is a particularly "precious" view of philosophy that seems to regard it as improper, or at best demeaning, for philosophy to concern itself with any tangibly practical question in the real world. This view would confine philosophy to the "pure" form, dealing only with those questions which are its exclusive preserve – and discarding "applied" philosophy in somewhat the same manner as "applied" science has sometimes been snubbed as a kind of problem-solving suitable for grease-besmeared mechanicals. Such a view (in either science or philosophy) can be regarded as socially objectionable; in the case of philosophy it seems also to rest on simple error. (Indeed, one feels that philosophers with so precious a view of their subject could probably benefit from trying to get out and about a bit more.) As Upton shows, the distinction between "pure" and "applied" philosophy is an illusion. Philosophy becomes "applied" simply when one or more of its usual and traditional enquiries are taken up for practical reasons, typically in the search for clarification of disputed terms in a practical debate.[12]

Having dismissed the "none of the above" view, it might still seem desirable for philosophy to confine itself to "medical meta-ethical" questions. This is because whilst those questions seem self-evidently philosophical, neither descriptive nor normative medical ethics questions lie within the philosopher's competence as such. This is true for descriptive medical ethics since in order to know who said what about which and when they said it, one needs the report of a competent observer and philosophers have neither training nor (often) interest in gathering observational data. And one might want to agree that philosophers ought to avoid trying to answer normative medical ethics questions with any kind of special "philosophical" authority.

Unfortunately the issue of philosophical involvement in normative medical ethics questions is much the most difficult of the three cases. This is because, in the first place, it is hard to tackle normative medical ethics questions without doing at least some philosophy, however informal, and in the second place, it is hard to tackle meta-ethical questions without giving comfort and succour to one side or the other in some practical, normative question. One cannot realistically endorse, for instance, a utilitarian approach to ethics without favouring the collective good over individual freedom of choice and this will impact upon debates concerning the decent limits of health promotion and other public health measures, such as vaccination or prenatal screening policies, or on the question of whether organ retrieval should be based on "opting in" or on "opting out". Those who, at the "meta-ethical" or theoretical level, urge the claims of individual duty against the claims of the collective good will also have an impact upon those debates, but generally in favour of the other side.

Moreover, the more intractable questions of moral judgement are typically entangled with questions of meaning and scope. This is evident in those most visible of medical ethics issues, such as whether and when abortion is permissible; whether we should withdraw feeding from the permanently comatose; and, nowadays, whether it could be legitimate to clone a human being. These ethical questions immediately precipitate questions of meaning and scope: respectively, when does human life begin or what is to count as human life? When does human life end? What is a person? What is justice, to whom does it apply, and how is it expressed in relation to the consumption of scarce healthcare resources? And so on.

Observations such as these are now fairly familiar, though not of course settled. At any rate, in holding a position on any of these normative questions one simply can't help having a position, willingly or otherwise, on the essentially philosophical questions with which they are entangled and it is philosophically obligatory to make one's own such underlying positions or presumptions transparent.

## Philosophy and medicine

There are other philosophical engagements bearing on reflection on ethical questions; these will, I trust, be recognisable in medical education, but maybe not always acknowledged as *philosophical*. For instance, key concepts in medicine, such as the nature and identity of health and illness, of normality, disease, and suffering, are not "given" in nature. Illnesses are not, as it were, self-labelling.

They involve a certain attitude towards things that we experience, a kind of agreement (which is often tied to a particular society) that something constitutes the kind of thing that excuses us from ordinary responsibilities, entitles us to special concern and consideration on the part of others, and so forth.

Some illness states involving acute pain, breathlessness, paralysis or fainting or so on might well be recognised as abnormal and fearsome in any culture. But other conditions that might be thought to constitute illnesses or diseases can vary between different cultures. Presymptomatic conditions disposing the "sufferer" to later pathology (for instance, obstruction of the coronary arteries) will be identified as such, and hence as disease states, only within societies concerned and able to diagnose them. And even here the picture is not a simple one; within the apparently similar societies of western Europe, Germans regard low blood pressure as a disease requiring treatment where British doctors regard low blood pressure as, if anything, a healthy sign.

It seems then that, in a very real sense, with regard to many conditions we do not so much *discover* as come to a kind of agreement about whether they will, in a certain context, be so disadvantageous or unwelcome as to constitute an abnormality, a disease or an illness. Where, moreover, do we draw the line between what falls inside and what falls outside the "normal" range? Blood pressure is an obvious example but so is the level and fluctuation of blood sugar, how much habitual consumption of a particular substance such as alcohol constitutes a pathological dependency, how restricted one's movements or faculties must be to be thought disabled or demented, and so on. The key distinction is between *descriptive* states of affairs in the world, that any competent observer ought to be able to pick out, and *normative* or *evaluative* judgements that some states of affairs are to be avoided and some are to be welcomed; this often depends on the circumstances in which observers find themselves. The distinction is a philosophical one and, whatever one might wish to call it, it is an essentially philosophical appreciation which acknowledges that we, rather than nature alone, supply the ideas and categories involved in picking out illness states from healthy states.[13]

This recognition invites a much broader philosophical interest in medicine. Reflections such as these invite us to think more generally about medicine's nature and goals, to which end one can then ask numerous and I think valuable particular questions. Here are some of them. Is medicine a science or an art? What kinds of knowledge and practice are constitutive of clinical medicine or of medical theory? What is the relationship between theory and experience in medicine? Clinical medicine involves *performance*; does it, or should it, involve *artistry* in any sense (and if so, in what sense)?[14, 15] What kinds of causes apply in medicine? Human beings vary in terms of how they get ill and how they respond to treatment. So how do statistical probabilities, derived from general populations of patients of a certain category, apply to individual treatment for specific patients?

In turn this requires us to think about how we should understand the human body. Is it a complicated kind of machine, an integrated closed system, the large-scale expression of molecular coding, an open, self-regulating system interacting with its environment, etc.? Or is it understood through distinct categories, incorporating psychological phenomena, biopsychosocial phenomena or the more elusive "embodied self".[16,17]

These are of course deep puzzles about our nature and our very essence. You would expect philosophers to be interested in such puzzles but perhaps it's less obvious that medicine's special kind of attention to the human body raises, inescapably, just these puzzles. Medicine is, however you look at it, simply bristling with philosophical puzzlement. Modern medicine raises the now-familiar ethical problems of when we should offer or withdraw treatment for fragile patients at the boundaries of life. This inevitably requires us to reflect on what constitutes the human person, on the nature of human experience and on the boundaries of the recognisably (or acceptably?) human. It requires us to consider the nature and importance of the will, particularly as genetic explanations are attempted for some antisocial behaviours, of decisions, of rationality, of individuals" own values and their personal goals.[18]

## Philosophy and the medical humanities

In Chapter 1 Greaves has described what we call the *integrated* conception of the medical humanities, in which the perspectives of the humanities and social sciences are to be incorporated alongside the perspectives of the natural sciences at the core of medical knowledge. Philosophy's interest in distilling and developing this conception of the medical humanities is a natural development from its interest in ethics in medicine. We can usefully regard the

attention to medical ethics, which perhaps came to the fore with
Ramsey's seminal call to regard the patient as a *person* in 1970,[19] as
a "herald" to draw our attention to a wider range of human values
that are at stake in the medical encounter. Ethics may be the first,
the most obvious, and even the most important of the human
values to be recognised in medicine but we can understand and
interpret those ethical values only by taking account of all the
human values important to the people involved. Though not all
equally important (or even necessarily relevant at all) in any given
clinical encounter, the human values generally at stake in clinical
medicine include:

- *aesthetic* values (such as the importance of appearance and
  normal functioning or of "body image"; the importance of
  elegance, economy, and even artistry in the physician's or the
  surgeon's practical interventions)
- *social* values (the expectations of conformity attending the roles
  and behaviours of both doctor and patient)
- *political* values (the requirements of co-ordinating the individual
  encounter within the institutional directives of organised
  healthcare – itself, in the United Kingdom, perhaps the most
  crucial remaining expression of solidarity)
- *intellectual* values (the mutual approach of different vocabularies
  on the part of patient and doctor in the search for effective and
  satisfying explanations and the doctor's search for theoretical
  economy and simplicity in those explanations as an expression
  of scientific method)
- and even *gustatory* values (the need to interest a recuperating
  patient in taking nourishment when it might be difficult for him
  or her to do so; or the need for children's treatment to be as
  palatable as possible in the interests of their compliance with it).

Philosophy is now recognising and considering this enlarged range
of values. In this sense, "philosophical medical humanities" in the
UK is comparable to that of "philosophical medical ethics" 20-odd
years ago. Although an important field of enquiry is recognisably
opening up, with philosophy as a catalyst, serious and sustained
explorations are only now beginning.[20]

The distinct humanities disciplines – history, the study of
literature, theology, anthropology, philosophy, and ethics, among
others – are, in their own right, forms of sustained enquiry into the
range of human experiences and the part played in shaping those

experiences by the wider range of human values. The medical humanities can bring together these enquiries in the special context of medical practice. In the process, I think we will come to appreciate how "medical understanding" itself becomes a way to understand ourselves as living, experiencing human selves. Now the habit of *critical reflection* – that is, thinking about the values and forms of knowledge appropriate to a particular subject – is a unifying feature of the humanities disciplines. But it is also the hallmark of philosophy as a discipline and to that extent philosophy occupies, I think, a pivotal place in the medical humanities.

## Medicine as a cultural good? A philosophical speculation

In much of this chapter I have been looking backward at the emergence of philosophy's role in the modern discourses of medical ethics and, in its current formulation, the newly crystallising enquiries of the medical humanities. Let me finish this chapter by looking forward. Newell and Gabrielson have suggested that the humanities are distinguished by their being concerned with "the human".[21] But it seems to me that this is to some extent true of all knowledge and all enquiry. In seeking to understand and control the world about us we are at the same time seeking to understand and affirm our own place within it. And this means seeking to understand *ourselves* a little better. In this sense the physical sciences, such as physics and chemistry – which enquire into the relationship between form and function, between the phenomena under observation and the nature and identity of the observation itself – are pursuing our self-understanding just as much as do the biological or even the behavioural sciences.

Of course, the emphases are different and it might even be (though I doubt it) that insights into our own nature as enquiring subjects are somehow "incidental" to the physical sciences where they are essential to the behavioural sciences. Be that as it may. The point is that all forms of enquiry may be capable of producing an *organising metaphor* under whose terms we will, for a period, fruitfully reconsider the narratives of our culture and of ourselves. Take the question of the freedom of the will. For western culture the architecture of theological speculation and the ideology of economic history have given us, through Manicheanism and Marxism respectively, organising metaphors of ourselves as corners of a cosmic battlefield contested by the forces of darkness and light or as the myriad minute gear-wheels of historical necessity. Psychoanalytic psychology, through Freud, and the molecular genetics that followed from Watson and Crick have also given organising metaphors of ourselves as matrices of unconscious desires or as somatic and behavioural expressions of our essential individual blueprints.

Modern biomedicine's inheritance is, in every sense, largely potentiated by the promise of disclosing the genetic influence over our life's course. In that sense it embodies the organising metaphor of molecular genetics in a particularly well-developed, well-modulated voice. It provides us with the modern form of the arena in which we examine our nature, our anxieties, our hopes, and our future potential. This is even more true now than it was when Byron Good pointed out the dominance of modern medicine over our suffering and our "salvation".[22] Many scholastic questions occupied philosophical enquiry for more than two millennia; for example, the freedom of the will, the relation between mind and body; the nature of consciousness, knowledge and judgement, the problem of personal identity, etc. Now, the "medical body", the body anatomised and reconstructed within the categories of biomedicine,[22] brings such questions urgently to life, giving them vivid, concrete, practical importance for perhaps the first time.[23]

Medicine and philosophy appear to share the same ambitious project of human self-understanding. Medicine concerns itself with the substance of our embodiment as selves and philosophy with the conceptual understanding of that embodiment. These two facets of our nature bespeak the perennial supposed "duality" of body and mind, matter and consciousness, with which we have too readily allowed ourselves to suppose that "the sciences" and "the humanities" are respectively concerned. Medicine and philosophy are, potentially, the first participants in a wider conversation between the sciences and the humanities. In this conversation, the modern gulf between those seemingly irreconcilable forms of knowledge, concerned respectively with the material world and the experiential world, can begin, tentatively, to be bridged.

# References and notes

1  Toulmin S. How medicine saved the life of ethics. In: de Marco JP (ed.). *New Directions in Ethics*. New York: Routledge and Kegan Paul, 1986; 265–81.
2  Davis JA. Whose life is it anyway? *BMJ* 1986; **292**:1128.

3   Downie R. The role of literature in medical education. *J Med Ethics* 1999; **25**: 529–31.
4   Scott PA. Imagination in practice. *J Med Ethics* 1997; **23**: 45–50.
5   General Medical Council. *Tomorrow's Doctors: recommendations on undergraduate medical education*. London: General Medical Council, 1993.
6   Collier JAB, Longmore JM, Hodgetts TJ. Fame, fortune, medicine and art. *The Oxford Handbook of Clinical Specialties*. Oxford: Oxford University Press, 1995: 413.
7   Lennon P. The guru and the gall. *The Guardian* 1992; 30 March: 23.
8   Raphael DD. *Moral Philosophy*. Oxford: Oxford University Press, 1981.
9   Greaves D. What are heart attacks? Rethinking some aspects of medical knowledge. *Med Health Care Philosophy* 1998; **1**: 133–41.
10  Gaarder J. *Sophie's World* (trans. P Møller). London: Phoenix, 1995.
11  Aristotle. *Politics* 1.9.1258a 10-14. In: Barnes J (ed.). *The Complete Works of Aristotle*. Princeton: Princeton University Press, 1984.
12  Upton H. Can philosophy legitimately be applied? In: Evans M (ed.). *Critical Reflection on Medical Ethics*. Stamford, CT: JAI Press, 1998: 123–38.
13  Canguilhem G. *On the Normal and the Pathological* (trans. CR Fawcett). New York: Urzone Inc., 1989.
14  Toulmin S. Knowledge and art in the practice of medicine: clinical judgement and historical reconstruction. In: Delkeskamp-Hayes C, Gardell Cutter MA (eds). *Science, Technology and the Art of Medicine*. Dordrecht: Kluwer Academic Publishers, 1993: 231–49.
15  Sacks O. *A Leg to Stand On*. London: Picador, 1984: see especially p.16.
16  Wulff HR. The disease concept and the medical view of Man. In: Querido A (ed.). *The Discipline of Medicine*. Amsterdam: Elsevier Science, 1994: 11–19.
17  Merleau-Ponty M. *Phenomenology of Perception* (trans. C Smith). London: Routledge and Kegan Paul, 1962.
18  Evans M. Pictures of the patient: medicine, science and humanities. In: Evans M, Sweeney K (eds). *The Human Side of Medicine*. London: Royal College of General Practitioners, 1998: 1–16.
19  Ramsey P. *The Patient as Person*. New Haven: Yale University Press, 1970.
20  Evans M, Greaves D. Exploring the medical humanities: a new journal will explore a new conception of medicine. *BMJ* 1999; **319**: 1216.
21  Newell JD, Gabrielson IW (eds). *Medicine Looks at the Humanities*. London: University Press of America, 1987: xvii.
22  Good B. *Medicine, Rationality and Experience*. Cambridge: Cambridge University Press, 1994: Chapter 3.
23  Evans M. The "medical body" as philosophy's arena. *Theoret Med Bioethics* 2000; **21**: in press.

# Alphabetical list of references

Aaron H. *Serious and Unstable Condition*. Washington DC: Brookings Institute, 1991

*Aberdare Leader* 1921; 19 November

Abse D. *Collected Poetry* London: Penguin, 1977

Ackerknecht EH. *Medicine at the Paris Hospital 1794–1848*. Baltimore: Johns Hopkins University Press, 1967

Adams RG, Allan G. *Placing Friendship in Context* Cambridge: Cambridge University Press, 1998

Allan G, Harrison K. *Placing Friendship in Context*. Cambridge: Cambridge University Press, 1998

Amenta M. Nurses as primary spiritual care workers. *Hospice J* 1988; **4**: 47–55

Anning S.T. A medical case book: Leeds, 1781–84. *Med History* 1984; **28**: 420–1

Anning ST. *The General Infirmary at Leeds*, 2 vols. Edinburgh and London: E and S Livingstone, 1963–6

Appleby G, Hunt L, Jacob M. *Telling the Truth About History*. New York: WW Norton, 1994

Aries P. *The Hour of Our Death*. New York: Alfred A Knopf, 1981

Aristotle. *Politics* 1.9.1258a 10-14. In: Barnes J (ed.). *The Complete Works of Aristotle*. Princeton, NJ: Princeton University Press, 1984

Aristotle. *Nicomachean Ethics*. New York: Random House, 1941:1097a-b

Aristotle. *Physics*. New York: Random House, 1941: Book II, Chapter 3

Arnold K. Birth and breeding: politics on display at the Wellcome Institute for the History of Medicine. In: Macdonald S (ed.). *The Politics of Display: museums, science, culture*. London: Routledge, 1998

Arnott R. Healing and medicine in the Aegean Bronze Age. *J Roy Soc Med* 1996; **89**: 265–9

Asbury JE, cited in Morgan DI (ed.). *Successful Focus Groups – advancing the state of the art*. London: Sage Publications, 1993

Asher R. The medical education of the patient and the public. In: Avery Jones F (ed.). *Talking Sense*. London: Churchill Livingstone, 1986

Ballard P, Finlay I, Searle C, Jones N, Roberts S. Spiritual perspectives among terminally ill patients: a Welsh sample. *Modern Believing* 2000; **41**(2): 30–8

Balmer J. *Sappho: Poems and Fragments*. Newcastle-upon-Tyne: Bloodaxe Books, 1992

*Barry Dock News*, 1921; 22 July

Bates ES (ed.). T*he Bible: designed to be read as living literature; The Old and New Testaments in the King James Version*. London: William Heinemann, 1936

*Bath Journal* 1751; 14 January

Beck U. *Risk Society: towards a new modernity* (trans. M Ritter). London: Sage, 1992

Becker MH. The health belief model and the sick role behaviour. *Health Education Monograph* **2**: 409–19

Belli A, Coulehan J (eds). *Blood and Bone: Poems by physicians*. Iowa City: Iowa Press, 1998

Benjamin W. *Illuminations*. New York: Schocken Books, 1969

Benson H. *Timeless Healing: the power and biology of belief*. London: Simon and Schuster, 1996

Bentley M. *Modern Historiography: an introduction*. London: Routledge, 1999

*Beowulf* (trans. M Alexander). Harmondsworth: Penguin, 1973

Berger J. *A Fortunate Man*. New York: Vintage Books, 1967

Berlin I. The apotheosis of the romantic will. In: *The Crooked Timber of Humanity*. London: Fontana Press, 1991

Berliner HS, Salmon JW. The holistic alternative to scientific medicine: history and analysis. *Int J Health Services* 1980; **10**: 133–47

Bevan H. *Records of the Salop Infirmary from the Commencement of the Charity to the Present Time*. Shrewsbury: Sandford and Howell, 1847

Bignell CJ. Chaperones for genital examination (editorial). *BMJ* 1999; **319**:137–8

Bolton G. A log fire warms you twice. *Lancet* 1997; **349**:1183

Bolton G. No thank you. *Lancet* 1997; **349**:217

Bolton G. Dregs. *Prog Palliat Care* 1997; **5**: 34

Bolton G. Every poem breaks a silence that had to be overcome;

the therapeutic power of poetry. *Feminist Rev* 1999; **62**: 118–33

Bolton G. *The Therapeutic Potential of Creative Writing*. London: Jessica Kingsley, 1999

Booth R, Stuart L. *My Kingdom of Books*. Talybont Ceredigion: Y Lolfa, 1999

Borsay, A. "Persons of Honour and Reputation": the voluntary hospital in an age of corruption. *Med History* 1991; **35**: 281–94

Borsay A. A middle class in the making: the negotiation of power and status at Bath's early Georgian General Infirmary, c.1739–1765. *Soc History* 1999; **24**: 269–86

Borsay A. An example of political arithmetic: the evaluation of spa therapy at the Georgian Bath Infirmary, 1742–1830. *Med History* 2000; **44**: 149–72

Borsay A. Cash and conscience: financing the General Hospital at Bath, c.1739–1750. *Soc History Med* 1991; **4**: 207–29

Borsay A. Returning patients to the community: disability, medicine and economic rationality before the Industrial Revolution. *Disabil Soc* 1998; **13**: 645–63

Borsay A. *Medicine and Charity in Georgian Bath: a social history of the general infirmary c1739–1830*. Aldershot: Ashgate, 1999

Boutall KA, Bozett FW. Nurses" assessment of patients' spirituality: continuing education implications. *Nurse Educ Today* 1993; **13**: 196–201

Boynton RS. The two Tonys. *New Yorker* 1997; 6 October

*British Medical Journal* 1892; 8 October: 787–8

*British Medical Journal* 1899; 23 September: 797

Broadie A. *The Scottish Enlightenment: an anthology*. Edinburgh: Canongate Classics, 1997

Brockbank W, Kenworthy F (eds). *The Diary of Richard Kay, 1716–51 of Baldingstone, near Bury: a Lancashire doctor*. Manchester: Chetham Society, 1968

Brody H. What does the primary care physician do that makes a difference? In: Stewart M (ed.). *Primary Care Research: traditional and innovative approaches*. Newbury Park, California: Sage Publications, 1991

Brook RH, Park RE, Winslow CM *et al*. Diagnosis and treatment of coronary disease: a comparison of doctors" attitudes in the USA and the UK. *Lancet* 1988; **189**: 750–3

Brown JH. *The Valley of the Shadow*. Port Talbot: Alun Books, 1981

Brown PS. The providers of medical treatment in nineteenth-century Bristol. *Med History* 1980; **24**: 313

Brunner E, Davey Smith G, Marmot M *et al*. Childhood social circumstances and psycho social and behavioural factors as determinants of plasma fibrinogen. *Lancet* 1996; **347**: 1008–13

Buer MC. *Health, Wealth, and Population in the Early Days of the Industrial Revolution*. London: George Routledge, 1926

Bunker JP. Ivan Illich and the pursuit of health. *J Health Service Res Policy* 1997; **2**: 56–9

Burnard P. Searching for meaning. *Nursing Times* 1988; **84**: 34–6

Burnett FH. *The Secret Garden*. Harmondsworth: Penguin, 1973

Bynum WF. Cullen and the nervous system. In: Doig A, Ferguson JPS, Milne IA, Passmore R (eds). *William Cullen and the Eighteenth-Century Medical World*. Edinburgh: University of Edinburgh Press, 1993

Byron C. Writers on teaching. In: Thomas S (ed.). *Creative Writing*. Nottingham: Nottingham University Press, 1995

Calman K, Downie R. Why arts courses for medical curricula? *Lancet* 1996; **347**: 1499–1500

Calman KC, Downie RS. Education and training in medicine. *Med Educ* 1988; **22**: 488–91

Campbell EJM. Basic science, science and medical education. *Lancet* 1976; **i**: 134–6

Campo R. *The Desire to Heal*. Norton: New York, 1997

Canguilhem G. *On the Normal and the Pathological* (trans. CR Fawcett). New York: Urzone Inc., 1989

Cannadine D. War and death, grief and mourning in modern Britain. In: Whaley J (ed.). *Mirrors of Mortality: studies in the social history of death*. London: Europa Publications, 1981

Capps LM. The memorial as symbol and agent of healing. In: Capps W (ed.). *The Vietnam Reader*. London: Routledge, 1991

Carey MA, cited in Morgan DI (ed.). *Successful Focus Groups – advancing the state of the art*. London: Sage Publications, 1993

Carr EH. *What is History?* Harmondsworth: Penguin, 1964

Cassell E. *The Nature of Suffering and the Goals of Medicine*. Oxford: Oxford University Press, 1991

Cawley N. An exploration of the concept of spirituality. *Int J Palliat Nurs* 1997; **3**: 31–6

Chalmers AF. *What is This Thing Called Science?* St Lucia, Queensland: University of Queensland Press, 1978

Charlton BG. Book review of Evidence-Based Medicine. *J Eval Clin Pract* 1997; **3**: 169–72

Cixons H. Writing as a second heart. In: Sellers S (ed.). *Delighting the Heart: A notebook by women writers*. London: The Women's Press

Clouser KD. Humanities and the medical school: a sketched rationale and description. *Br J Med Educ* 1971; **5**: 226–31

Cohen S. Psychosocial models of the role of social support in the etiology of physical disease. *Health Psychol* 1988; **7**: 269–97

Cohen S. Social ties and susceptibility to the common cold. *JAMA* 1997; **277**: 1940–1

Collier JAB, Longmore JM, Hodgetts TJ. Fame, fortune, medicine and art. *The Oxford Handbook of Clinical Specialties*. Oxford: Oxford University Press, 1995

Conrad LI, Neve M, Nutton V, Porter R, Wear A. *The Western Medical Tradition 800 BC to AD 1800*. Cambridge: Cambridge University Press, 1995

Cook S. Religion. In: Hastings J (ed.). *Encyclopaedia of Religions and Ethics*, vol X. Edinburgh: T and T Clark, 1918

Corin E. The social and cultural matrix of health and disease. In: Evans RG, Barer ML, Marmor TR (eds). *Why are Some People Healthy and Others Not?* New York: Aldine De Gruyter, 1994

Cornette K. Forever I am weak, I am strong. *Int J Hospice Palliat Nurs* 1997; **3**: 1

Cronin AJ. *The Citadel*. London: Gollancz, 1937

Culler J. *Literary theory*. Oxford: Oxford University Press, 1997

Curl JS. *A Celebration of Death*. London: Constable, 1980

Curtis P. The Whitehall Cenotaph: an accidental monument. *Imperial War Museum Rev* 1994; **9**: 31–41

Davenport C. *Heredity in Relation to Eugenics*. USA: Henry Holt, 1911

Davies J. War Memorials. In: Clark D (ed.). *The Sociology of Death*. Oxford: Blackwell, 1993

Davies W (ed.). *Dylan Thomas*. London: JM Dent, 1997

Davis JA. Whose life is it anyway? *BMJ* 1986; **292**: 1128

Dear M (ed). *The Power of Geography: how territory shapes social life*. Boston: Unwin Hyman, 1989

Declaration of Windsor. In: Philipp R, Baum M, Mawson A, Calman KC. *The humanities in medicine: beyond the millennium*. London. The Nuffield Trust, 1999

Department of Health. *Saving Lives: Our healthier nation*. London: HMSO, 1999

Dickens C. *Hard times*. Bradbury & Evans, 1854

Dixon M, Sweeney KG, Pereira Gray DJ. The physician-healer: ancient magic or modern science? *Br J Gen Pract* 1999; **49**: 309–13

Dominian J. The doctor as a prophet. *BMJ* 1983; **287**: 1925–7

Donaldson L. *Stem Cell Research: medical progress with responsibility.* London: Department of Health, 2000

Dostoyevsky F. *The Idiot* (trans. D Magarshack). Harmondsworth: Penguin Classics, 1955

Downie R (ed.). *The Healing Arts.* Oxford: Oxford University Press, 1994

Downie R. The role of literature in medical education. *J Med Ethics* 1999; **25**: 529–31

Downie R, Macnaughton J. Should medical students read Plato? *Med J Aust* 1999; **170**: 125–7

Downie R, Macnaughton J. *Clinical Judgement: evidence in practice.* Oxford: Oxford University Press, 2000

Drever F, Whitehead M. *Health Inequalities.* London: Office for National Statistics, 1997

Dunthorne H. *The Enlightenment.* London: Historical Association, 1991

Dyson J, Cobb M, Forman D. The meaning of spirituality: a literature review. *J Adv Nurs* 1997; **26**: 1183–8

Eagleton T. *The Illusions of Postmodernism.* Oxford: Blackwell, 1996

Edassey D, Kuttierath SK. Spirituality in the secular sense. *Eur J Palliat Care* 1998; **5**: 165–7

Edwards RHT. Time for sharing responsibility. *J Roy Coll Physicians London* 1999; **33**: 145–7

Eisenberg DM, Davis RB, Ettner SL *et al.* Trends in alternative medicine use in the United States, 1990–1997: results of a follow-up national survey. *JAMA* 1998; **280**: 1569–75

Eliot G. *Daniel Deronda.* London: Blackwood, 1876

Eliot G. *The Mill on the Floss.* London: Blackwood, 1860

Eliot TS. *Collected Poems (The Four Quartets).* London: Faber, 1936: 189–223

Ellis C. The old, the sick and the poor. In: Ellis C (ed.). *Mid Victorian Sleaford 1851–1871.* Lincoln: Lincolnshire Library Service, 1981

Elsdon R. Spiritual pain in dying people: the nurse's role. *Prof Nurse* 1995; **10**: 641–3

Elstad JI. The psycho-social perspective in social inequalities in health. *Sociol Illness Health* 1998; **20**: 698–718

Elton GR. *The Practice of History.* London: Collins, 1969

Engelhardt HT Jnr. *The Foundations of Bioethics.* Oxford: Oxford University Press, 1986

Epstein RM. Mindful practice. *JAMA* 1999; **282**: 833–9

Evans D. Pro-attitudes to pre-embryos. In: Evans D (ed.).

*Conceiving the Embryo.* The Hague: Martinus Nijhoff, 1997

Evans M. Human individuation and moral justification. In: Evans D (ed.). *Conceiving the Embryo.* The Hague: Martinus Nijhoff, 1997

Evans M. The "medical body" as philosophy's arena. *Theoret Med Bioethics* 2000; **21**: in press

Evans M, Greaves D. Exploring the medical humanities: a new journal will explore a new conception of medicine. *BMJ* 1999; **319**: 1216

Evans M, Sweeney KG. *The Human Side of Medicine.* Occasional Paper 76. London: Royal College of General Practitioners, 1998

Evans M, Greaves D, Pickering N. Medicine, the arts and imagination (correspondence). *J Med Ethics* 1997; **23**: 254

Evans RJ. *In Defence of History.* London: Granta, 1997

Farquhar G. *The Beaux' Stratagem.* London: A and C Black, 1998

Feynman RP. *The Meaning of It All.* London: Allen Lane, 1998

Fido R, Pott M. Using oral histories. In: Atkinson D, Jackson M, Walmsley J (eds). *Forgotten Lives: exploring the history of learning disability.* Kidderminster: British Institute of Learning Disabilities, 1997

Finlay IG, Maughan TS, Webster DJT. Portfolio learning: a proposal for undergraduate cancer teaching. *Med Educ* 1994; **28**: 79–82

Finlay IG, Maughan TS, Webster DJT. A randomised controlled study of portfolio learning in undergraduate cancer education. *Med Educ* 1998; **32**: 172–6

Firth R. *Elements of Social Organization.* London: CA Watts, 1951

Fishbein M, Azjen B. *Belief, Attitude, Intention and Behavior.* New York: Wiley, 1975

Fissell ME. The disappearance of the patient's narrative and the invention of hospital medicine. In: French R, Wear A (eds). *British Medicine in an Age of Reform.* London: Routledge, 1991

Fletcher C, Peeling P. *Talking and Listening to Patients: a modern approach.* London: Nuffield Provincial Hospitals Trust, 1988

Fontanarosa PB, Lundberg GD. Alternative medicine meets science. *JAMA* 1998; **280**: 1618–19

Forster EM. *Howard's End.* Harmondsworth: Penguin Books, 1969

Foucault M. *Discipline and Punish: the birth of the prison* (trans. A Sheridan). Harmondsworth: Penguin, 1977

Foucault M. *The History of Sexuality,* 3 vols (trans. R Hurley). Harmondsworth: Penguin, 1981

Foucault M. *The Birth of the Clinic: an archaeology of medical perception* (first published 1963) (trans. AM Sheridan). London: Routledge, 1989

Foundation for Integrated Medicine. *Integrated Healthcare: a way forward for the next five years?* London: Prince of Wales Initiative on Integrated Medicine, 1997

Fox R. The evolution of American bioethics. Paper given to the Welsh Section of the British Sociology Association Medical Sociology Group in Swansea on 1 May 1997

Frankl VE. *Man's Search for Meaning*, 5th edn. London: Hodder & Stoughton, 1987

Freud S. Thoughts for the times on war and death. In: Strachey J, Freud A (eds). *The Standard Edition of the Complete Psychological Works of Sigmund Freud*, vol.XIV, 1914–1916. London: Hogarth Press, 1957

Gaarder J. *Sophie's World* (trans. P Møller). London: Phoenix, 1995

Gaffney A. *Poppies on the up-platform: commemoration of the Great War in Wales*. Thesis. Cardiff: University of Wales Press, 1996

Gaffney A. *Aftermath: Remembering the Great War in Wales*. Cardiff: University of Wales Press, 1998

Galton F. *Memoirs of My Life*. London: Methuen, 1908

Garattini S, Garattini L. Pharmaceutical prescriptions in four European countries. *Lancet* 1993; **342**: 1191–2

General Medical Council. *Tomorrow's Doctors: recommendations on undergraduate medical education*. London: General Medical Council, 1993

General Medical Council. *Proposals for Revalidation*. London: General Medical Council, 2000

*Gentleman's Magazine*. A View of the Many Peculiar Advantages of Public Hospitals. 1741; **XI**: 476–7

George D, Hirnshall H. *My Heart Soars*. Saanichton BC: Hancock House, 1974

Giddens A. *Modernity and Self-Identity: self and society in the late modern age*. Cambridge: Polity Press, 1991

Gillon R. Imagination, literature, medical ethics and medical practice. *J Med Ethics* 1997; **23**: 3–4

Gillon R. Welcome to medical humanities – and why (editorial). *J Med Ethics* 2000; **26**: 155–6

Glover J. *Humanity: a moral history of the twentieth century*. London: Jonathan Cape, 1999

Glymour C, Stalker D. Engineers, cranks, physicians, magicians. *N Engl J Med* 1983; **308**: 960–4

Goffman E. *Relations in Public*. Harmondsworth: Allen Lane,

Penguin Press, 1971

Goffman E. *The Presentation of Self in Everyday Life.* New York: Doubleday Anchor Books, 1959

Good B. *Medicine, Rationality and Experience.* Cambridge: Cambridge University Press, 1994

Goodman A. *The Street Memorials of St Albans Abbey Parish.* St Albans: St Albans and Hertfordshire Architectural and Archaeological Society, 1987

Gordon C (ed.). *Michel Foucault power/knowledge: selected interviews and other writings 1972–1977.* Brighton: Harvester, 1980

Gorer G. The pornography of death. In: *Death, Grief and Mourning in Contemporary Britain.* London: Cresset Press, 1965

Gott T (ed.). *Don't Leave Me This Way: art in the age of AIDS.* Canberra: National Gallery of Australia,1994

Graham-Pole J. In: Belli A, Coulehan J (eds). *Blood and Bone: Poems by physicians.* Iowa City: Iowa Press, 1998

Graham-Pole J. Children, death and poetry. *J Poetry Therapy* 1996; **9**: 129–41

Greaves D. What are heart attacks? Rethinking some aspects of medical knowledge. *Med Health Care Philosophy* 1998; **1**: 133–41

Greenberg A. Lutyens' Cenotaph. *J Soc Architectural Historians* 1989; **48**: 5–23

Greenhalgh T. Writing as therapy: effects on immune mediated illness need substantiation in independent studies. *BMJ* 1999; **319**: 270–1

Greenhalgh T, Hurwitz B. Why study narrative? *BMJ* 1999; **318**: 48–50

Gregory A. *The Silence of Memory.* Oxford: Berg, 1994

Grene M. *The Knower and the Known.* Berkeley: University of California Press, 1974

Grey A. The spiritual component of palliative care. *Palliat Med* 1994; **8**: 215–21

Gropper C. Well versed in medical practice. *Lancet* 1998; **353**: 759

Guthrie D. *A History of Medicine.* London: T Nelson and Sons, 1945

Haldane D, Loppert S. *The Arts in health care: learning from experience.* London: King's Fund, 1999

Hall B. Spirituality in terminal illness: an alternative view of theory. *J Holistic Nurs* 1997; **15**: 82–96

Hall PA. Social capital in Britain. *Br J Political Sci* 1999; **29**:417–61

Hamberger R. Quoted in Bolton G. *The Therapeutic Potential of Creative Writing: Writing myself.* London: Jessica Kingsley, 1999

Hamberger R. Acts of Parking. *New Statesman* 1995; 24 November: 49

Hamberger R. *Warpaint Angel* Leicester: Blackwater Press, 1997

Hamilton D. Believing in patient's beliefs: physician attunement to the spiritual dimension as a positive factor in patient healing and health. *Am J Hospice Palliat Care* 1998; **15**: 276–9

Hammond JL, Hammond B. *The Bleak Age* (first published 1934). West Drayton: Penguin, 1947

Hampshire S. *Innocence and Experience*. London: Allen Lane, 1989

Hampton JR. The end of medical history? *J Roy Coll Physicians London* 1998; **32**: 366–75

Handerin T. *The Oxford companion to philosophy*. Oxford: Oxford University Press, 1995

Hansler D, Cooper C, cited in Nyamathia A, Shuler P. Focus group interview: a research technique for informed nursing practice. *J Adv Nurs* 1986; **15**: 128–88

Harris J. *The Value of Life*. London: Routledge and Kegan Paul, 1985

Hay M. Principles in building spiritual assessment tools. *Am J Hospice Care* 1989; **8**: 25–31

Hazelgrove J. *Spiritualism and British Society Between the Wars*. Manchester: Manchester University Press, 2000

Heath I. Uncertain clarity: contradiction, meaning and hope. William Pickles Lecture. *Br J Gen Pract* 1999; **49**: 651–7

Heath I. *The Mystery of General Practice*. London: Nuffield Hospitals Provincial Trust, 1995

Helleiner KF. The vital revolution reconsidered. *Can J Economics Political Sci* 1957; **XXIII**: 6

Higgs E, Melling J. Chasing the ambulance: the emerging crisis in the preservation of modern health records. *Soc History Med* 1997; **10**: 127–36

Hilliard N. Spirituality in hospice care. *Palliat Care Today* 1998; **6**: 52–3

*Hippocratic Writings* (trans. GER Lloyd). London: Penguin, 1950

Hodges I, Norton V. *Artists at Stewart Villa*. Wellington, New Zealand: Department of Health, 1991

Hollinger R. *Postmodernism and the Social Sciences: a thematic approach*. Thousand Oaks, California: Sage, 1994

Homberger E. The story of the Cenotaph. *Times Literary Supplement* 1976; 12 November: 1429–30

Honderich T. *The Oxford Companion to Philosophy*. Oxford: Oxford University Press, 1995

Human Genetics Advisory Commission. *Cloning Issues in Reproduction, Science and Medicine*. London: HGAC, 1998

Hunt SM, McEwen J, McKenna SP. *Measuring Health Status*. London: Croom Helm, 1986

Huppauf B. War and death: the experience of the First World War. In: Crouch M, Huppauf B (eds). *Essays on Mortality*. Sydney: University of New South Wales, 1985

Ibsen H. *An Enemy of the People*. London: Eyre Methuen, 1980

Illich I. *Limits to medicine. Medical Nemesis: the expropriation of health*. Harmondsworth: Penguin Books, 1976

Inglis KS. War memorials: ten questions for historians. *Guerres Mondiales et Conflits Contemporains* 1992; **CLXVII**: 5–21

Jackson M. Images of deviance: visual representations of mental defectives in early twentieth-century medical texts. *Br J History Sci* 1995; **28**: 319–37

Jackson M. Medical humanities in medical education. *Med Educ* 1996; **30**: 396

Jackson M. The use of historical study in medical research. *Fam Pract* 1996; **13** (suppl 1): 17–20

Jacobi J. *The Psychology of CG Jung*, 7th edn. London: Routledge and Kegan Paul, 1968

Jenkins K. *Re-Thinking History*. London: Routledge, 1991

Jewson ND. Medical knowledge and the patronage system in eighteenth-century England. *Sociology* 1974; **8**: 371–2

Jewson ND. The disappearance of the sick man from medical cosmology, 1770–1870. *Med History* 1976; **10**: 227–30

Jha SR. The tacit-explicit connection: Polanyian integrative philosophy and a neo-Polanyian medical epistemology. *Theoretical Med Bioethics* 1998; **19**: 547–68

Jonas WB. Alternative medicine – learning from the past, examining the present, advancing the future. *JAMA* 1998; **280**: 1616–18

Jones R. patients' attitudes to chaperones. *J Roy Coll Gen Pract* 1985; **35**: 192–3

Jones RH. The use of chaperones by general practitioners. *J Roy Coll Gen Pract* 1983; **33**: 25–6

Kelley A. *Poetry Remedy*. Newmill: Hypatia Trust, 1999

Kernick D, McDonald R. What is health economics and why do Primary Care Groups need to get to grips with it? In: Sweeney KG, Dixon M (eds). *The Emergence of Primary Care Groups: from rhetoric to reality*. Oxford: Radcliffe Medical Press, 2000

Kessler S. Invited essay on the psychological aspects of genetic counselling. V. Preselection: a family coping strategy in

Huntingdon's disease. *Am J Med Genet* 1988; **31**: 617–21

Kessler S, Bloch M. Social systems responses to Huntington's disease. *Fam Process* 1989; **28**: 59–68

Kevles DJ. *In the Name of Eugenics: genetics and the uses of human heredity.* New York: Alfred A Knopf, 1985

King A. *Memorials of the Great War in Britain. The Symbolism and Politics of Remembrance.* Oxford: Berg, 1998

Kirklin D. *Public consultation on human cloning begins: an opportunity to examine the role of pro-attitudes in the embroy research debate and their effect on legislation.* MA Thesis. London: Kings's College, 1998

Kleinman A. *Writing at the margin: discourse between anthropology and medicine.* Berkeley: University of California Press, 1995

Kolb D, Rubin IM, McIntyre JM. *Organisational behaviour: an experiental approach.* Englewood Cliffs: Prentice-Hall, 1994

Kopelman LM. Bioethics and humanities: what makes us one field? *J Med Philosophy* 1998; **23**: 356–68

Kumar K. *From Post-Industrial to Post-Modern Society: new theories of the contemporary world.* Oxford: Blackwell, 1995

Labun E. Spiritual care: an element in nursing planning. *J Adv Nurs* 1990; **13**: 314–20

Laidlaw R. The Gresford disaster in popular memory. *Llafur* 1995; **VI**: 123–46

Lakoff G, Johnson M. *Metaphors We Live By.* Chicago: University of Chicago Press, 1980

Langer SK. *Feeling and Form.* London: Routledge and Kegan Paul, 1953

Laurillard D. *Rethinking Teaching.* London: Routledge, 1993

Le Fanu J. The fall of medicine. *Prospect* 1999; **July**: 28–31

Lennon P. The guru and the gall. *The Guardian* 1992; 30 March: **23**

Leonard P. *Postmodern Welfare: reconstructing an emancipatory project.* London: Sage, 1997

Lieven M. *Senghennydd: The Universal pit village, 1890–1930.* Llandysul: Gomer Press, 1994

Lloyd DW. *Battlefield Tourism. Pilgrimage and the Commemoration of the Great War in Britain, Australia and Canada, 1919–1939.* Oxford: Berg, 1998

Lock S, Wells F (eds). *Fraud and Misconduct in Medical Research,* 2nd edn. London: BMJ Books, 1996

Longley E. The Rising, the Somme and Irish memory. In: Ni Dhonnchadha M, Morgan T (eds). *Revising the Rising.* Londonderry: Field Day, 1991

Longworth P. *The Unending Vigil. A History of the Commonwealth War Graves Commission 1917–1984*. London: Leo Cooper, 1985

Loudon I (ed.). *Western Medicine: an illustrated history*. Oxford: Oxford University Press, 1997

Loudon I. *Medical Care and the General Practitioner 1750–1850*. Oxford: Clarendon Press, 1986

Lyon D. *Postmodernity*. Buckingham: Open University Press, 1994

Mabek CE, Olesen F. Metaphorically transmitted diseases: how do patients embody medical explanations? *Fam Pract* 1997; **14**: 271–8

Macnaughton J. The humanities in medical education: context, outcomes and structures. *J Med Ethics: Med Humanities* 2000; **26**: 23–30.

Margotta R. *The Hamlyn History of Medicine*. London: Reed International, 1996

Marinker M. The clinical method. In: Cormach J, Marinker M, Morrell D (eds). *Teaching Clinical Method*. London: Kluwer Medical, 1981

Markus T. *Buildings and Power: freedom and control in the origin of modern building types*. London: Routledge, 1993

Marmot MG *et al*. Health inequalities among British civil servants: the Whitehall II study. *Lancet* 1991; **337**: 1387–93

Marteau T, Richards M (eds). *The Troubled Helix*. Cambridge: Cambridge University Press, 1996

Marwick A. *The Nature of History*. London: Macmillan, 1970

Matarasso F. *Defining Values: Evaluation in the Arts*. Stroud: Comedia, 1996

Matarasso F. *Poverty and Oysters: The Social Impact of Local Arts Development in Portsmouth*. Stroud: Comedia, 1998

Matarasso F. *Regular Marvels: A Handbook for Animateurs, Practitioners and Development Workers in Dance, Mime, Music and Literature*. Leicester: Community Dance and Mime Foundation, 1994

Matarasso F. *Use or Ornament? The Social Impact of Participation in the Arts*. Stroud: Comedia, 1997

Maudsley H. In: McDougal J (ed.). *Theatres of the Body*. London: Free Association Books, 1989

McGouran R. What price prevention? *Hospital Doctor* 1997; April 3: 12

McKee DD, Chappel JN. Spirituality and medical practice. *J Fam Pract* 1992; **35**: 201–8

McKeown T. A sociological approach to the history of medicine.

*Med History,* 1970; **14**: 342

McManus IC. Humanity and the medical humanities. *Lancet* 1995; **346**: 1143–5

McSherry W, Draper P. The debates emerging from the literature surrounding the concept of spirituality as applied to nursing. *J Adv Nursing,* 1998; **27**: 683–91

Merleau-Ponty M. *Phenomenology of Perception* (trans. C Smith). London: Routledge and Kegan Paul, 1962

Mickley J, Soeken J, Belcher A. Spiritual well-being: religiousness and hope among women with breast cancer. *Image: J Nursing Scholarship* 1992; **24**(4): 267–72

Mill JS. On liberty (1859): In: Warnock M (ed.) *Utilitarianism.* Glasgow: Collins, 1962

Millison M, Dudley JR. Providing spiritual support: a job for all hospice professionals. *Hospice J* 1992; **8**(4): 49–65

Mitchell A, McCormack M. *The Therapeutic Relationship in Complementary Health Care.* London: Churchill Livingstone, 1998

Molière JB. *The Imaginary Invalid* (trans. J Wood). Harmondsworth: Penguin, 1959

Montgomery SM, Bartley MJ, Wilkinson RG. Family conflict and slow growth, *Arch Dis Child* 1997; **4**: 326–30

Moriarty C. Christian iconography and First World War memorials. *Imperial War Museum Rev* 1992; **6**: 63–75

Moriarty C. The absent dead and figurative First World War Memorials. *Trans Ancient Monuments Soc* 1995; **39**: 7–40

Moriarty G. *Taliruni's Travellers: an arts worker's view of evaluation.* Stroud: Comedia, 1997

Mumford L. *The Myth of the Machine, the Pentagon of Power.* New York: Harcourt, Brace, Jovanovich, 1970

Munslow A. *Deconstructing History.* London: Routledge, 1997

Muntaner C *et al.* The social class determinants of income inequalities and social cohesion. *Int J Health Services.* 1999; **29**(4): 699–732

Narayanasamy A. Nurses' awareness and education preparation in meeting their patients' spiritual needs. *Nurse Educ Today* 1993; **13**: 196–201

National Council for Hospice and Specialist Palliative Care Services. *Specialist Palliative Care: a statement of definitions.* Occasional Paper 8. London: National Council for Hospice and Specialist Palliative Care Services, 1995

Naylor CD. Grey zones of clinical practice: some limits to evidence based medicine. *Lancet* 1995; **345**: 840–2

Newell JD, Gabrielson IW (eds). *Medicine Looks at the Humanities.* London: University Press of America, 1987

NHS Wales. *Putting patients First.* Cardiff: Welsh Office, 1998

Noble J. General internal medicine in internal medicine: at the core or on the periphery? *Ann Intern Med* 1992; **116**: 1058–60

Nochlin L. *Realism.* Harmondsworth: Penguin, 1971

Nowell-Smith PH. *Ethics.* Harmondsworth: Penguin, 1954

Oldnall A. A critical analysis of nursing: meeting the spiritual needs of patients. *J Adv Nurs* 1996; **23**: 138–44

Pahl R. *On Friendship.* Cambridge, Polity Press, in press

Pellegrino ED. Educating the humanist physician. An ancient ideal reconsidered. *JAMA* 1974; **227**: 1288–94

Pellegrino ED. *Humanism and the Physician.* Knoxville: University of Tennessee Press, 1979

Pellegrino ED. Introduction. In: Belli A, Coulehan J (eds). *Blood and Bone: Poems by physicians.* Iowa City: Iowa Press, 1998

*Penarth News* 1924; 13 November

Pendleton D, Hasler J. *Doctor-patient Communication.* London: Academic Press, 1983

Pennebaker JW, Kiecott Glaser J, Glaser R. Disclosure of traumas and immune function: health implications for psychotherapy. *J Consult Clin Psychol* 1988: **56**: 239–45

Pereira Gray DJ. Nakedness in medicine. In: Pereira Gray DJ (ed.). *The Medical Manual.* Bristol: Wright, 1986

Peters RS. *The Concept of Education.* London: Routledge and Kegan Paul, 1967

Peterson MJ. *The Medical Profession in Mid-Victorian London.* Berkeley: University of California Press, 1978

Petherbridge D, Jordanova L. *The Quick and the Dead.* London: SouthBank Centre, 1997

Philo C. "Enough to drive one mad": the organization of space in nineteenth-century lunatic asylums. In: Wolch J, Dear M (eds). *The power of geography: how territory shapes social life.* Boston: Unwin Hyman, 1989: 258–90

Piaget J. *Structuralism* (trans. C Maschler). New York: Harper and Row, 1970

Piehler GK. The War Dead and the Gold Star: American commemoration of the First World War. In: Gillis JR (ed.) *Commemorations: the politics of national identity.* Princeton: Princeton University Press, 1994

Piles C. Providing spiritual care. *Nurse Educator* 1990; **15**: 36–41

Plato. *Republic.* London: Sphere Books, 1970: Book X

Polanyi M. *Personal Knowledge.* London: Routledge and Kegan Paul, 1958

Polanyi M. *The Tacit Dimension.* London: Routledge and Kegan Paul, 1967

Polanyi M. Tacit knowing: its bearing on some problems of philosophy. In: Grene M (ed.). *Knowing and Being.* London: Routledge and Kegan Paul, 1969

Polanyi M, Prosch H. *Meaning.* Chicago: University of Chicago Press, 1975

Porter D. The mission of social history of medicine: an historical overview. *Soc History Med* 1995; **8**: 345–8

Porter D, Porter R. *Patient's Progress: doctors and doctoring in eighteenth-century England.* Cambridge: Polity Press, 1989

Porter R. *The Enlightenment.* Basingstoke: Macmillan, 1990

Porter R (ed.). *The Cambridge Illustrated History of Medicine.* Cambridge: Cambridge University Press, 1996

Porter R. *The Greatest Benefit to Mankind: a medical history of humanity from antiquity to the present.* London: HarperCollins, 1997

Portes A. Social capital: its origins and applications in modern sociology. *Ann Rev Sociol* 1998; **24**: 1–24

Quereshi B. Muslim patients and the British general practitioner. In: Pereira Gray DJ (ed.). *The Medical Manual.* Bristol: Wright, 1984

Radcliffe Richards J. *Human Nature after Darwin.* London: Routledge, 2000

Rael EGS *et al.* Sickness absence in the Whitehall II study, London: the role of social support and material problems. *J Epidemiol Comm Health* 1995; **49**: 474–81

Ramsey P. *The Patient as Person.* New Haven: Yale University Press, 1970

Raphael DD. *Moral Philosophy.* Oxford: Oxford University Press, 1981

Reed P. An emerging paradigm for the investigation of spirituality in nursing. *Res Nursing Health* 1992; **15**: 349–57

Reese WD, Lutkins SG. The mortality of bereavement. *BMJ* 1967; **4**: 13–16

Reilly DT, Taylor MA, McSharry C, Aitchinson T. Is homeopathy a placebo response? A controlled trial of homeopathic immunotherapy (HIT) in atopic asthma. *Complement Therap Med* 1993; **1**: 24–5

Risse G. *Hospital life in Enlightenment Scotland: care and teaching at the Royal Infirmary of Edinburgh.* Cambridge: Cambridge University Press, 1986

Risse G.B. Medicine in the age of enlightenment. In: Wear A (ed.). *Medicine in Society: historical essays.* Cambridge: Cambridge University Press, 1992

Roberts JAF. *An Introduction to Human Genetics,* 2nd edn. Oxford: Oxford University Press, 1959

Roddie B. Coming to terms with death. *BMJ* 1999; **317**: 1737

Rolfe IE, Andren JM, Pearson S, Hensley MJ, Gordon JJ. Clinical competence of interns. *Med Educ* 1995; **29**: 225–30

Ross L. The nurse's role in assessing and responding to patients' spiritual needs. *Int J Palliat Nurs* 1997; **3**: 37–45

Roter DL. Patient Participation in the Provider Patient Interaction. *Health Educ Monograph,* 1977; **5**: 281–315

Royal College of General Practitioners. *The Future General Practitioner: learning and teaching.* London: British Medical Association, 1972

Sabovic Z, Pearson D (eds). *A Healthy Heritage: collecting for the future of medical history – Conference proceedings.* London: Wellcome Trust, 1999

Sackett DL, Haynes RB, Tugwell P. *Clinical Epidemiology: a basic science for clinical medicine.* Boston: Little, Brown, 1985

Sackett DL, Richardson WS, Rosenberg W, Haynes RB. *Evidence-Based Medicine. How to learn and Teach EBM.* New York: Churchill Livingstone, 1997

Sacks O. *A Leg to Stand On.* London: Picador, 1984

Sacks O. *The man who mistook his wife for a hat.* London: Picador, 1985

Sarason BR *et al. Social Support: an interactional view.* Chichester: John Wiley, 1990

Sarup M. *An Introductory Guide to Post-Structuralism and Postmodernism,* 2nd edn. Hemel Hempstead: Harvester Wheatsheaf, 1993

Sawday J. *The Body Emblazoned.* London: Routledge, 1995

Schlink B. *The Reader* (trans. Janeway CB) London: Phoenix House, 1997

Schmidt HG, Machiels-Bongaerts M, Hermans H, ten Cate TJ, Venekamp R, Boshuizen HPA. The development of diagnostic competence: comparison of a problem-based, an integrated, and a conventional medical curriculum. *Acad Med* 1996; **71**: 658

Scott D. *Michael Polanyi.* London: SPCK, 1996

Scott PA. Imagination in practice. *J Med Ethics* 1997; **23**: 45–50

Seale C. The evaluation of health care. In: Davey B, Popay J (eds). *Dilemmas in Health Care*. Milton Keynes: Open University Press, 1993

Secretary of State for Health. *A First Class Service*. London: Department of Health, 1998

Shakespeare W. *Hamlet*

Shakespeare W. *The Tempest*

Shaw GB. *The Apple Cart*. Harmondsworth: Penguin, 1946

Shaw GB. *The Doctor's Dilemma: A Tragedy*. Harmondsworth: Penguin, 1946

Sherrin N. *The Oxford Dictionary of Humorous Quotations*. Oxford: Oxford University Press, 1995

Shorter E. *From Paralysis to Fatigue: a history of psychosomatic illness in the modern era*. New York: Freedom Press, 1992

Simpsen B. Nursing the spirit. *Nursing Times* 1998; **84**: 31

Singer P (ed.). *Embryo Experimentation: ethical, legal and social implications*. Cambridge: Cambridge University Press, 1990.

Skrabanek P. *The Death of Humane Medicine*. London: Social Affairs Unit, 1994

Smith BH. Old malady. *JAMA* 1995; **274**: 1412

Smyth JM, Stone AA, Hurewitz A, Kaeu A. Effects of writing about stressful experiences on symptom reduction in patients with asthma or rheumatoid arthritis. *JAMA* 1999; **281**: 1304–9

Snow CP. *The Two Cultures and the Scientific Revolution*. The Rede Lecture. Cambridge: Cambridge University Press, 1959

Social Exclusion Unit. *National Strategy for Neighbourhood Renewal: a framework for consultation*. London: Cabinet Office, 2000

Southgate B. *History: what and why? Ancient, Modern and Postmodern Perspectives*. London: Routledge, 1996

Sparrow F. *Through the Large Glass*. London: London College of Printing, 1997

Spiegel D. Healing words: emotional expression and disease outcome (editorial). *JAMA* 1999; **281**: 1328–9

Steiner G. *In Bluebeard's Castle: some notes towards the re-definition of culture*. London: Faber and Faber, 1971

Stenhouse L. *An Introduction to Curriculum Research and Development*. London: Heinemann, 1975

Stevens A. Recording the history of an institution: the Royal Eastern Counties Institution at Colchester. In: Atkinson D, Jackson M, Walmsley J (eds). *Forgotten Lives: exploring the history of learning disability*. Kidderminster: British Institute of Learning Disabilities, 1997

Stiles WB. Verbal response modes and dimensions of interpersonal roles: a method of discourse analysis. *J Personal Social Psychol* 1978; **36**: 693–703

Sweeney KG. Evidence and uncertainty. In: Marinker M (ed.). *Sense and Sensibility in health care.* London: BMJ Books, 1996

Sweeney KG, MacAulay D, Pereira Gray DJ. Personal significance: the third dimension. *Lancet* 1998; **351**: 134–6

Szreter S. The importance of social intervention in Britain's mortality decline c.1850–1914: a re-interpretation of the role of public health. *Soc History Med* 1988; **1**: 1–37

Tarlow S. *Bereavement and Commemoration: an archaeology of mortality.* Oxford: Blackwell, 1999

Taylor EJ. Amenta M, Highfield M. Spiritual care practices of oncology nurses. *Oncol Nurs Forum* 1995; **22**: 31–9

Taylor EJ, Amenta M. Midwifery to the soul while the body dies: spiritual care among hospice nurses. *Am J Hospice Palliat Care* 1994; **11**: 28–35

Thomas KB. *Religion and the Decline of Magic.* London: Weidenfeld and Nicolson, 1971

Thomas KB. The temporary dependant patient. *BMJ* 1974; **1**: 59–61

Thompson EP. *The Making of the English Working Class.* Harmondsworth: Penguin, 1963

Thomson M. *The Problem of Mental Deficiency: eugenics, democracy and social policy in Britain c.1870–1959.* Oxford: Clarendon Press, 1998

Tilley N. *After Kirkholt: theory, method and results of replication evaluations.* London: Home Office, 1993

Tolstoy L. *The Death of Ivan Illyich and other stories* (trans. R Edmonds). Harmondsworth: Penguin, 1960

Toon P. *What is Good General Practice?* Occasional Paper 65. Exeter: Royal College of General Practitioners, 1994

Toon P. *Towards a Philosophy of General Practice: a study of the virtuous practitioner.* Occasional Paper 78. London: Royal College of General Practitioners, 1999

Tosh J. *The Pursuit of History: aims, methods and new directions in the study of modern history,* 2nd edn. London: Longman, 1991

Toulmin S. How medicine saved the life of ethics. In: de Marco JP (ed.). *New Directions in Ethics.* New York: Routledge and Kegan Paul, 1986

Toulmin S. Knowledge and art in the practice of medicine: clinical judgement and historical reconstruction. In: Delkeskamp-Hayes

C, Gardell Cutter MA (eds). *Science, Technology and the Art of Medicine*. Dordrecht: Kluwer Academic Publishers, 1993

Townsend C. *Vile Bodies*. Munich New York: Prestel, 1998

Toynbee A. *Lectures on the Industrial Revolution of the Eighteenth Century in England* (first published 1884). London: Longmans, Green and Co., 1913

Traill HD, Mann JS. *Social England*, 7 vols. London: Cassell, 1895

Treuherz J. *Hard Times: social realism in Victorian art*. London: Lund Humphries and New York: Moyer Bell, in association with Manchester City Art Galleries, 1987

Uchino BA *et al*. The relationship between social support and physiological processes: a review with emphasis on underlying mechanisms and implications for health. *Psychol Bull* 1996; **119**: 488–531

University of Wales College of Medicine. Prospectus for A104 and A106 courses, 2000–2001

Upton H. Can philosophy legitimately be applied? In: Evans M (ed.). *Critical Reflection on Medical Ethics*. Stamford, CT: JAI Press, 1998

Vernon PE (ed.). *Creativity*. Harmondsworth: Penguin, 1970

Walter T. Developments in spiritual care of the dying. *Religion* 1996; **26**: 353–63

Walter T. War grave pilgrimage. In: Reader I, Walter T (eds). *Pilgrimage in Popular Culture*. London: Macmillan, 1993

Warren J. *The Past and its Presenters: an introduction to issues in historiography*. London: Hodder and Stoughton, 1998

Wear A (ed.). *Medicine in Society: historical essays*. Cambridge: Cambridge University Press, 1992

Weiss JM, Sunder S. Effects of stress on cellular immune responses in animals. *Rev Psychiat* 1992; **11**: 145–80

*Wellcome News* Hidden evidence: sudden death and antipsychotics. 1999; **18**: 20

*Wellcome News* Aberdeen anguish: the Aberdeen typhoid outbreak of 1964. 1999; **18**: 16–17

Wellcome Trust. *Response to the HGAC/HFEA Consultation on Cloning Issues in Reproduction, Science and Medicine*. London: Wellcome Trust, 1998

Whorton JC. Traditions of folk medicine in America. *JAMA* 1987; **257**: 1632–5

Wilde O. *The Picture of Dorian Gray*. London: Minster Classics, 1968

Wilkinson M. *Creative Writing: Its role in evaluation*. London: King's Fund Publishing, 1999

Wilkinson RG. *Unhealthy Societies*. London: Routledge, 1996

Williams R. *Monmouth Diocesan Newsletter* 1998; **121**: 5

Williams R, Jones D. *The Cruel Inheritance*. Pontypool: Village Publishing, 1990

Willis J. *The Paradox of Progress*. Oxford: Radcliffe Medical Press, 1995

Winchester S. *The Surgeon of Crowthorne*. London: Penguin, 1998

Winter JM. *The Great War and the British People*. London: Macmillan, 1986

Winter JM. *Sites of Memory, Sites of Mourning: the Great War in European cultural history*. Cambridge: Cambridge University Press, 1995

Woodward J. *To Do the Sick No Harm: a study of the voluntary hospital system to 1875*. London: Routledge and Kegan Paul, 1974

World Library. *The Bible: a multimedia experience*. Irvine, California: Softkey, 1995

Wulff HR. The disease concept and the medical view of Man. In: Querido A (ed.). *The Discipline of Medicine*. Amsterdam: Elsevier Science, 1994

Zola E. *Dr Pascal*. Stroud: Alan Sutton Publishing, 1989

# Index

Note: Figures in **bold** refer to figures; those in *italic* to tables and boxed material

Abbeyville Community Cemetery, France 180
Aberdare, south Wales 183
Aberdeen typhoid outbreak 67
abortion debate 115–16
Abse, Dannie 128, 157
Acton, Lord JEE 51–2, 54
Aesclepian traditions 96
aesthetic appreciation 230
alternative medicine 58–9, 237
analysis, philosophical 253
anatomy teaching 170
Anderson, Betsy 157
*Angela's Ashes* 157
antihypertensive therapy 227
*The Apple Cart* 245
"archetypes 239
argument analysis 194, 206
Aristotle 212–13, 215
Armistice 177
art
    death portrayed in 171
    defining 37–8
    doctor-patient relationship in 61–2, 193
    relationship with health 39
    *see also Dance of Death*
arts and health 246–7
    expressions of 153–4, 187–8
    relationship to medical humanities 188–90
    *see also* arts and health projects; community arts projects; creative writing; poetry
arts and health projects
    art:health relationship 39
    costs/negative impacts of 44–5
    defining art 37–8

defining health 38–9
evaluation 9–10, 36–7, 48
    impact *v* value 42–3
    indicators and methods 46
    interpretation of results 47
    need for 41–2
    reporting back 47–8
    goals 39–40
    planning 45–6
    principles for 43–4
    relationship of medical humanities 188–90
    types of practice 40–1
asthma 132
authors, medically-trained 168
*Awakenings* 158

bad news consultation 127–8
Bala, north Wales 182
Barber-Surgeons Company 58
Barthel Index 38
basal cell carcinoma 157
Bauby, Jean Dominique 157
Bedingfield, James 65
bedside medicine 10–11, 58–9, 61–2
*The Bell Jar* 157
Benjamin, Walter 170
bereavement
    effects on terminally ill 141
    in Great War 177–8
    mortality associated with 96
    portrayal in arts 193
Berger, John 200
Bible 243–5, 246
Bichat, Marie Francois Xavier 60
bioethics 21
    *see also* medical ethics
Blake, William 172–3

body image 161
*Body Mask* 174
Bohr, Nils 98
brain surgery 128
Breakwell, Ian 151, 169, 171
  *Body Mask* 174
  *Death Masks* 174
  *Deathrap* 173–4
  *Death's Dance Floor* 151, 169
  *The Rose* 172–3
breast cancer
  family theories of inheritance 104–5
  impact of diagnosis 93–4
  mastectomy 61–3
  patient's poetry 123
breast examination 93–4
Bristol Infirmary 65
*British Medical Journal* 127
British Society for the History of
  Medicine 52
Brunonians 228
Buckell, Lindsay 131
Buckle, HT 51–2
Burnett, Frances Hodgson 246
Burney, Fanny 62

Cadoxton Boys' School, Barry 183
Cain, Eleanor 182
cancer patient
  "heroic" surgery 11, 62–3
  impact of diagnosis 93–4
  interpersonal relationships 142–3
  poetry written by 121–3
*Cancer Ward* 158
*Candour* 127–8
*carpe diem* 169, 170
Carr, EH 54
Cartesian dualism 95–6
case histories, in arts 157–8, 191–3,
  236, 243–6
cemeteries 169–70, 179–80
Cenotaph, London 178
chaperones 94
chaplain 139, 145
children
  bad news consultation 127–8
  death 157
Christianity 130–40
*The Citadel* 163, 245
clinical significance 87
clinical trials 132, 226–8
coercive healthism 91
Comedia 189
common (or community) activities
  32–3, 239, 242–3, 247
communication skills 163–4, 193,
  205–6, 236, 240–2
communities
  attitudes to death 169–70

notions of 8–9, 25, 30
  war memorials 152–3
community arts projects 9, 187–8, 189
*Compendium of Cases from the Bristol
  Infirmary* 65
*The Compleat Angler* 243–4
connections 206
consultation 78, 83–98
  analyses of 83
  disingenuousness in 88–91
  and healthcare rationing 91–2
  interpretation of narrative 84–6,
    205–6
  philosophy of medical practice 95–7
  physical examination 92–5
  Rubik's cube analogy 83–4, 97–8
  use of medical evidence 87–8, 89
  *see also* doctor-patient relationship
coronary heart disease 32, 89–90
counselling
  genetic 106–8
  in terminal illness 145
"counterculture", to medicine 14–15,
  154, 195–6
creative writing 80, 120–1, 131, *see also*
  poetry
Crickhowell, south Wales 183–4
critical judgement 195
critical reflection 8, 67–8, 261
Cronin, AJ 163, 245
Cullen, William 60
cultural advantage 30–2

da Vinci, Leonardo 157
dance 239
*The Dance of Death* 169–71, 174–6
  *Death Masks* 174
  *Deathrap* 173–4
  *The Rose* 172–3
Dante 172
Davies, John 182
death
  addressed in poetry 123
  artworks concerned with 171
  attitudes to 169–70
  undergraduate's experience of
    151–2
  *see also* bereavement; mortality; *The
    Dance of Death*
*The Death of Ivan Illyich* 246
*Death Masks* 174
*Deathrap* 173
*Death's Dance Floor* 151, 169
*Decline and Fall of the Roman Empire* 51
depression
  poetry written in 125–6
  portrayal in the arts 157, 192–3
descriptive medical ethics 255, 256
designer babies 112

diagnosis
  impact of 93–4
  patient narrative 65–6, 84–6, 205–6
Dickens, Charles 224
disingenuousness 88–91
dissecting room 170
*Divine Comedy* 172
*The Diving Bell and The Butterfly* 157
*The Doctor* 61–2, 193
*Doctor Jekyll and Mister Hyde* 163
doctor-patient relationship
  18th-19th century 10–11, 65–6
    and medical knowledge 59–60
    and medical marketplace 57–9
    and medical practice 61–4
    portrayal in art 61–2, 193
  *see also* consultation
doctors
  approach to death 170
  authors 168
  "educated" 194–5, 225–6
  humanity/compassion in 190–1,
    204–5, 225
  intervention strategies 89–90, 91
  poetry written by 126–8
  prescribing habits 90
  reputation/image of 91, 167–8, 245
  role of self 89–90
  thinking/reasoning 89
  *see also* consultation; doctor-patient
    relationship
*The Doctor's Dilemma* 245
Dostoyevsky, Feodor 116
dozenepil 91
drama 163–4, 193, 208
drug prescription 90, 91–2
dualism 95–6, 262
Dunn, Douglas 193
Durham Cathedral 172

Eckersley, Kitty 182
"educated" doctors 194–5, 225–6
Einstein, Albert 245
Eliot, George 109–10, 233
Elton, GR 54
embryo research 112–14
embryo screening 102, 110–12
emotions
  awareness of 209
  communication of 240–3
  expression in arts 209, 236
empiricism 51–2, 54, 228
*The Enemy of the People* 245
*The English Patient* 157
Enlightenment 50–1, 95–6
*Erin Brockovich* 158
ethics, *see* medical ethics
Ethics in Medicine SSM 199
eugenics 110–12

*Everyman* 233–4
evidence-based medicine (EBM) 87,
    132, 223–4
  evaluation of evidence 88, 193–4,
    206
  nature of evidence 87, 90, 226–7
  reinterpretation for personal care
    238
  relevance to individuals 90, 227–8,
    237–8

"facts" 224–5
faith 224–5, 243–4
family
  attitudes to death 170
  notions of 9, 26–7, 28
  of terminally ill 144
  theories of disease inheritance
    104–6
  value of 201, 207
Fanconi's anaemia 110–11
farming communities 28–9
Fawcett's Pills 59
fear 136, 145, 157
figurative knowledge 86
Fildes, Sir Luke 61–2, 193
film 158, 208
First World War, *see* Great War
*Fly On, My Sweet Angel* 157
Forster, EM 200, 206
*A Fortunate Man* 200
French Revolution 51
Freud, Sigmund 175–6
friendship 9, 27
  amongst hospice patients 142
  in culturally advantaged 30–2
  promotion of 32–3
  and well-being 32, 34
  in the young 34–5
  *see also* personal communities
funeral ritual 179

Galloway, Janice 193
Galton, Francis 111
Geesin, Ron 172, 173
General Medical Council (GMC) 66,
    156–7, 164–5, 191, 194–6, 198
genetic counselling 106–8
genetic revolution 101–3
  Human Impact SSM 201
  legacy of eugenics 110–12
  philosophical dimensions 262
genetic testing 79, 102
  counselling 106–8
  family interpretations of 79, 104–6
  impact of self-knowledge 104
  perceptions of risk 106
  receiving results 108–9
Gibbon, Edward 51

GMC, *see* General Medical Council
Government White Papers 188
Graham-Pole, John 127–8
graveyards, *see* cemeteries
Great War
  gravestone inscriptions 179–80
  local community memorials 178–9
  loss of life in 177–8
  national memorials 178
  non-repatriation of bodies 178
Gregory, Professor John 190–1
Grocer's Company 58
*gwerin* 242

Hahnemannians 228
*Hard Times* 224
Harvey, William 59–60
Hay Literary Festival 247
health
  inequalities of 24, 188–9
  meanings of 9–10, 38–9, 96–7
  nature and identity of 257–8
  social determinants of 8–9, 23–4,
    96, 188–9
health care rationing 91–2
Health Education Authority (HEA)
  29–30
health indices 38–9
heredity 101, 103–4
"heroic" surgery 11, 62–3
Hey, William 64
Hill, Christopher 52
history 10
  intellectual development of 50–7
  philosophy of 16–17, 54–7
  value of study 193–4, 239
*History of the Civilisation of England*
  51–2
history of medicine 10–11, 50, 52
  doctor-patient relationship 65–6
  medical knowledge 59–60
  medical marketplace 57–9
  medical practice 61–4
  relevance to contemporary practice
    66–8
  value of study 194
Hobsbawm, Eric 52
holism 59
holistic care 136–7
Holman, Margaret 124
Holme Tower Marie Curie Centre
  140–5
Holy Scripture 243–5, 246
hope 143
hospice 137
  Christian basis of 139–40
  patients' poetry 121–3
  patients' views of spiritual care
    140–5

hospice chaplain 139, 145
hospital model of medicine 10–11, 58,
  60, 65–6
hospitals, 18th-19th century 63–5
Hoult, Mr G 182
*Howard's End* 206
human cloning debate 112–16
Human Fertilisation and Embryology
  Act (1990) 114
Human Fertilisation and Embryology
  Authority (HFEA) 113–14
Human Genetics Advisory
  Commission (HGAC) 113–14
Human Genome Project 102
Human Impact of the Genetic
  Revolution (SSM) 201
human nature 1–2
human self-understanding 254, 261–2
human values 8, 260
humanistic perspectives 16–17, 207
humanities 2
  meaning of 15–16
  relevance to health 246–7
  *see also* medical humanities
humanity 190–1, 204–5, 225
humoralism 59–60, 68
humour 141
Huntington's disease 107
Hygeian traditions 96–7
hymns 145
hypochondriasis 246
hypothetico-deductive reasoning 89
hysterical conversion disorders 246

Ibsen, Henrik 245
illness, nature of 257–8
*The Imaginary Invalid* 246
imagination 98, 193, 200–1, 245
Imperial War Graves Commission 178,
  181
induction principle 89
indwelling 230–1
inherited disease 104–6, *see also* genetic
  testing
intellectual passions 231
*The International Herald Tribune* 111
intuitive deductive thinking 89
ISIS-2 trial 226–7

James, Henry 193
*Jane Eyre* 157
*Journal of the American Medical
  Association* 127
Jung, Carl 239

Kafka, Franz 157
Kahlo, Frida 158
Kantianism 98
Kay, Dr Richard 62–3

kin links 26–7
knowledge
    indwelling 230–1
    nature of 229–32
    personal 232–4
    tacit 229–30
    verification of facts 231–2

*The Lancet* 126, 127

language
    use in cloning debate 112–16
    use in patient narrative 86, 205–6
    use in relation to embryo screening
        111–12
Larkin, Philip 193
*Last Orders* 158
Leeds Infirmary 64
Lewis, CS 193
life, prolongation of 85–6
literature 239
    healthcare issues in 245
    intrinsic value of 195–6
    as source of human experiences
        157–8, 191–3, 236, 243–6
    writers with medical training 168
Literature and Medicine SSM 162–3
Llangollen International Musical
    Eisteddfod 247
longevity, value of 85–6
*Love Story* 158
Luton, social support in 29–30

McKeown, Thomas 53
*The Magic Mountain* 158
Mahler, Gustav 158
*The Making of the English Working Class*
    52
*The Man Who Mistook His Wife for a
    Hat* 158
Mann, Thomas 158
'manner', of doctors 190–1
Marx, Groucho 85
Marxist historiography 52
mass media 111–12, 184
mastectomy 61–3
medical arts 19–22
medical education
    admission criteria 165, 175, 191
    affective aspects 225–6
    cognitive aspects 225
    communications skills teaching
        163–4
    community placements 161–2
    creative arts in 175
    ethics teaching 13, 21, 190, 206
    GMC recommendations 156–7,
        191, 196, 198
    oncology teaching 160–1

postgraduate 187
    sexuality awareness teaching 162
    teaching methods 191
    *see also* medical humanities,
        undergraduate courses
medical ethics
    philosophical questions 255–7
    teaching of 13, 21, 190, 206
medical history, *see* history of medicine
*Medical Humanities* 213, 247
medical humanities 3, 7, 19–21, 153–4
    ends and means of 212–16
    instrumental values 20, 191–2
        argument construction 194, 206
        communication skills 163–4,
            193, 205–6, 236, 240–2
        evaluation of evidence 193–4,
            206
        joint investigation 210
        sources of human experience
            157–8, 191–3, 236, 243–6
    nature and conception of 1–3, 7–8,
        13–19, 154, 259–61
    non-instrumental values 192,
        194–7, 212–16
        "counterculture" to medicine
            14–15, 154, 195–6
        development of broad
            perspectives 207
        development of understanding
            207–8
        education 194–5, 225–6
        humanity 190–1, 204–5, 225
        recreation/relaxation 19–20
        self-awareness 195, 209
    place of philosophy 259–61
    postgraduate courses 187
    and social role of medicine 20–1
    undergraduate courses 156–7, 187
        additive 196, 197–8
        aims of 154
        complementary 200–2
        evaluation of 154–5, 164–5, 204,
            210–12
        integrative 199–200
        justification of 191–7
        portfolio learning 152
medical interventions
    cultural influences 89–90
    imposition of 91
    rationing 91–2
medical knowledge 223–5
    18th–19th century 59–60
    resources for 1–2
medical marketplace 57–9
medical records 11, 61–4, 66–7
medical student
    experience of death 151–2
    selection criteria 165, 191

medicine
  bedside model 10–11, 58–9, 61–2
  "crisis" in 7, 13, 91, 167–8, 245
  hospital model 10–11, 58, 60, 65–6
  nature and goals of 14, 252, 258–9
  philosophy of 16–17, 95–7, 251–4
  social role of 20–1
  see also history of medicine
The Meeting 123
memorials 152–3
memories, shared 241–2
Meno 229
mental disorder
  examples in literature 157, 192–3, 246
  poetry written in 125
meta-ethics 255, 256–7
Metamorphosis 157
metaphors 86, 125–6
metre 130
Mexican Day of the Dead 173
Mill, JS 195, 209
mind-body relations 1, 95–6, 230, 262
mining accidents 178–9
Moliere, JBP 246
moral imagination 193
moral judgement 257
moral sensitivity 207
Morgan, Alexander 65
Morgangni, Giovanni Battista 60
mortality
  18th-19th century healthcare 64
  following bereavement 96
  see also death
Morton, Angela 125–6
Munchausen's syndrome 246
Muriel 121–3
music 145, 239
musician 216

narrative, see patient narrative
National Eisteddfod of Wales 239, 242, 247
National Health Service (NHS) 91–2, 98
National Institute of Clinical Excellence (NICE) 92
neighbours 27
neurological disability 157
neurology 232
new genetics, see genetic revolution
Newton, Sir Isaac 60
NHS, see National Health Service
NHS Wales 240
NICE, see National Institute of Clinical Excellence
normative medical ethics 255, 256–7
Nottingham Health Profile 38–9

occupational communities 25
On Liberty 195
oncology teaching 160–1
operational knowledge 86
oral histories 11, 66–7
Osler Club of London 52
outcome evaluation 36, 48

paediatrics 127–8
pain
  patients' attitudes to 11, 62–3
  somatic 80, 120, 137
painting, process of 214–15
paintings 61–2, 193
papeles picados 173
parkinsonism 158
patient narrative
  demise of 10–11, 65–6
  interpretation of 84–6, 205–6
"patient-centred" care 190–1
Peace Day Celebrations 178
Penarth, south Wales 182
Pennington, Professor Hugh 67
personal communities 9, 26
  changes in time 28–9
  in culturally advantaged 30–2
  family 26–7, 28
  friends and neighbours 27, 34–5
  mapping of 27–8
  promotion of 32–4
  and well-being 32, 34
personal development 133, 195
personal identity 93–4
personal knowing 226, 228–9, 231, 232–4
Personal Knowledge 228
personal and professional development (PPD) modules 199–200
personal significance 88
personhood debate 115–16
Philadelphia 158
philosophers 250
philosophy
  authentic problems of 250, 253–4
  and human self-understanding 254, 261–2
  instrumental forms of 253
  and medical ethics 255–7
  of medical practice 16–17, 95–7, 251–4
  nature and goals of medicine 252
  nature and identity of illness 257–8
  pure v applied 256
philosophy teaching 193–4, 199, 201, 239
physical examination 92–5
The Picture of Dorian Gray 245–6
Plath, Sylvia 156, 193
Plato 201, 207–8, 229

poetry 80, 119
  communication through 124–6
  death addressed in 123
  evaluation of students' 211–12
  form of 129–30
  from hospice patient 121–3
  introducing to patients 132–3
  and personal development 120–1, 133
  portrayal of illness and suffering 157
  therapeutic benefits 132
  written by doctors 126–8
Polanyi, Michael 228–34
Political Philosophy SSM 201
political power 56–7
Popper, Karl 245
portfolio learning 152, 158–60
positivism 95–6
postgraduate medical education 187
postmodernism 54–6
Potter, Denis 157
power 56–7
PPD modules, see personal and professional development modules
pro-attitudes 115–16
professional reflexivity 8, 67–8, 261
Progress in Palliative Care 127
psoriasis 157
psychology 232
Pulsford, William 63
Putting Patients First 240

quality of life 85–6

Rain Man 158
Ranke, Leopold von 51
rationing, health care 91–2
reasoning 89
religion 139–40, 145, 224–5, 243–4
Republic 201, 207–8
revalidation 164–5
rheumatoid arthritis 132
rhyme 130
Richards, Martin 105
ritual 144, 179, 180
Roddie, Betty 123
Rogers, Lambert 128
role play 163–4, 193
The Rose 172–3
rose windows 172
Royal College of Physicians 58
Royal College of Surgeon of England 58
Royal Free and University College Medical School 201
Royal Society of Medicine 52

Sacks, Oliver 8, 17, 158

Saving Lives: our Healthier Nation 188
Schlink, Bernard 36, 48
science, definition 37
Scientific Revolution 60
Scottish Society for the History of Medicine 52
sculpting 164
sculpture 181
The Secret Garden 246
self, role of 89–90
self-awareness 195, 209
self-esteem 33
self-understanding 254, 261–2
Senghennydd pit explosion, south Wales 178–9
sexuality
  awareness teaching 162
  and physical examination 94–5
Shaw, Bernard 245
siblings 26, 28
The Sick Rose 172–3
sickle cell disease 108
sildenafil 91
simile 122
The Singing Detective 157
social advantage 24, 30–2
social capital 29–30
Social Capital and Health 29
social convoy 28–9
social determinants of health 8–9, 23–4, 96, 188–9
social history 51–2
social history of medicine 52–3
social inequalities 24, 188–9
social networks
  correlation with health 8–9, 23–4, 34
  promotion of 32–4
  studies of 25–6
  see also friendship; personal communities
society, role of medicine in 20–1
Society for the Social History of Medicine 52–3
Solzhenitsyn, Alexander 158
somatisation 80, 120, 137
special study modules (SSMs)
  additive courses 197–8
  complementary courses 200–1, 207
  Ethics in Medicine 199
  Human Impact of the Genetic Revolution 201
  integrative courses 199
  Literature and Medicine 162–3
  Political Philosophy 201
spirituality
  ambiguity in health care 137–9
  concepts of 137–8, 141
  hospice patients' perspectives 140–5

and religion 139–40
spouse 144
SSMs, *see* special study modules
statistical significance 87, 227–8
stigmatisation 142–3
streptokinase 226–7
stress 96
*The Surgeon of Crowthorne* 246
surgery
    18th-19th century 62–4
    poetry about 128
Swift, Graham 158
*Synopsis Nosologiae Methodicae* 60
syphilis 157

taboo 171
tacit integration 232
tacit knowledge 229–30
theatrical techniques 163–4
thermography 174
Thomas, Dylan 157–8, 246
Thompson, Edward 52
*The Times* 111–12
*To Kill a Mocking Bird* 157
Tolstoy, Leo 246
*Tomorrow's Doctors* 66, 156–7, 191,
    194–5
total pain 137
tragedies 152–3, 184–5
transferrable skills
    argument analysis 194, 206
    communication 163–4, 193, 205–6,
      236, 240–2
    evidence assessment 88, 193–4, 206
*Troilus and Cressida* 157
*The Troubled Helix* 105
tuberculosis 157, 158
Twain, Mark 246

University of Wales College of
    Medicine
    community medicine placement
      161–2
    Literature and Medicine SSM
      162–3
    oncology project 160–1
    portfolio learning project 158–60

sexuality awareness teaching 162

Viagra (sildenafil) 91
Vietnam War memorials 184
virtue ethics 96
visual arts 61–2, 157–8, 193, 208
Voltaire 167
voluntary hospitals 63–4

Wales
    community cultural activities 239,
      242–3, 247
    hospice patients 141–5
    mining accidents 178–9
    sustainable health plans 247
    war memorials 182, 183
Walton, Izaak 243–4
war 152–3, 175–6
war memorials 153, 184–5
    Great War
      civic pride in 183–4
      committees 180–2
      local community 178–9, 180
      physical forms of 181
      unveiling ceremonies 182–3
    Vietnam war 184
Webster, Charles 53
"well-being" 10
*What the poem means* 124
wheel windows 172
Whitehall Study 24
Wilde, Oscar 245–6, 250
*Winnie the Pooh* 157
women 180–3
Women's Institutes 33
work 34–5
Worshipful Society of Apothecaries 52
writing
    creative 80, 120–1, 131
    physical act of 124
writing skills 205
Wyper, Private James 180

young people 34–5

Zola, Émile 101, 103–4, 116